SURVIVING CANCER

SURVIVING CANCER

by Dee Simmons

Harrison House
Tulsa, Oklahoma

05 04 03 02 01   10 9 8 7 6 5 4 3 2 1

Surviving Cancer

ISBN 1-57794-391-0
Copyright © 2001 by Dee Simmons
Ultimate Living International, Inc.
P.O. Box 191326
Dallas, TX 75219

Published by Harrison House, Inc.
P.O. Box 35035
Tulsa, Oklahoma 74153

To My Daddy

William Henry Gee

Beloved father, godly example, wonderful teacher, and forever friend. Daddy taught me the books of the Bible at an early age, led me in the prayer for my salvation, spanked me for my mischievous habits, and put cardboard in his shoes so mother could buy dresses for me. Thank you for loving our mother, my sister Sandra, my brother James, and me, and for your uncompromising devotion to our Lord. I am so happy that you encouraged me to write this book and lived to see it completed.

To Charlotte Hale

The friendship and encouragement you have given me has made a significant impact on my life. Thank you for being such a rare treasure and inspiration in my life.

Acknowledgments

I wish to thank the many cancer survivors, their families, and various distinguished medical institutions and doctors whose wisdom, medical research, and personal stories are included in this book. In particular, special thanks to the American Cancer Society, Cancer Treatment Centers of America in Tulsa, The University of Texas M.D.

Anderson Cancer Center in Houston and its President and eminent cancer researcher, John Mendelsohn, M.D.

Thoughtful and generous help was provided by Richard Howe, Ph.D., retired President of Pennzoil and a tireless advocate for prostate cancer research, and his wife Dee; Philanthropist Michael Milken, who founded and heads CaP CURE, devoted to facilitating research and cures for prostate cancer; Frieda Courson of Atlanta and her husband Tom; author/producer Susan Wales and her daughter Megan Chrane; singer Destinae Rae; prostate cancer activist Tom Redmond, retired CEO of the Aussie hair care products company; Anne Platz, Atlanta interior designer and author; former Miss America, Cheryl Salem, who with her husband, Harry, devotes her life to full-time Christian ministry; and to the countless others whose stories appear here anonymously. We know who you are and are so grateful for the many heartfelt and sensible suggestions by those who have "been there".

And, to my very dear friend and physician, Dr. George Peters, Executive Director of The University of Texas Southwestern Center for Breast Care, who helped me wage my battle against breast cancer with the best medical care and advice possible.

Special thanks to Lou Ann York, my friend and publicist, who spent many hours pulling loose ends together in order to meet deadlines.

My thanks and deep gratitude, also, to the extraordinary efforts and involvement of everyone at Harrison House Publishers. Your devotion to excellence and accuracy is inspiring, as is your hope that future cancer survivors may find some measure of comfort and courage within these pages.

And, lastly, to my good friend and First Lady of Oral Roberts University, Lindsay Roberts, who has been my shining example of "faith, hope and optimism".

Table of Contents

FOREWORD

Dee Simmons is a cancer survivor who has thought long and hard about how to deal with the issues that confront cancer patients and their loved ones. She has drawn on her own experiences and those of many other patients to create a vision of how to redirect one's focus, how to draw upon one's internal strengths and the help of friends, how to find the best professional advice, and how to cope with this unwelcome and disturbing event. She offers many sound ideas that have come from her thoughtful consideration of what it means to have cancer.

Dealing with cancer requires effective treatment by an expert physician. Mrs. Simmons describes how a patient can become a participant in this process, how selecting a course of therapy can be a learning experience that empowers a patient with knowledge and clarifies inherent uncertainties. She gives guidance on how to draw upon human and spiritual resources to regain control and to face the future with the greatest possible hope. Cancer patients and their families and friends will be grateful for the inspired and forthright counseling Dee Simmons offers.

Cancer is a shocking, life-changing event. All those "normal" daily worries and activities are abruptly replaced by the need to make decisions on complicated treatment options. Dealing with uncertainty becomes a way of life. Unfortunately, for many types of cancer, optimal therapy is still a matter of research rather than a well-standardized formula. And, although the majority of cancer patients can expect an outcome that is successful in eliminating the disease, many patients must face the fact that there is a risk of recurrence or are forced to deal with a prolonged illness.

Cancer patients experience a loss of control in ways that our ordinary experiences may not prepare us for. For many, I think *Surviving Cancer* will provide significant help on the road to recovery.

John Mendelsohn, M.D.
President
The University of Texas M.D. Anderson Cancer Center

PREFACE

This is the book I wish someone had placed in my hands on March 10, 1987, when I first heard the words *infiltrating ductile carcinoma.* Like many others who learn they have cancer, I had little idea of what to expect. None of my friends had experienced cancer, and in those days few people even discussed the subject.

What I wanted then was the sort of practical advice, born of experience, that you'll find in these pages: advice from men and women of every age, background, race, and type of cancer, even some deemed incurable, who survived and today are going strong.

During the fourteen years since my own cancer recovery, I have counseled with thousands of men, women, and children with various forms of the disease. My Rolodex bulges with names of patients, doctors, treatment centers, research scientists, and other resources.

A lot of what I learned about cancer is told here through the experiences of numerous other patients who, like me, plotted individual strategies for survival. We learned to team up with our doctors and therapists. We read. We listened. We became proactive, and blessedly, we survived.

These people are winners. Perhaps they didn't know they would be on D-Day (diagnosis day), when their lives took such an abrupt, unfair, and nasty turn. Perhaps like me, who at age forty-seven learned I had breast cancer, they started out ignorant of the battles ahead. Maybe they wondered about some things. How will this change me? My career? My relationships? What about my future? (Will I even have a future?) Am I really up to this challenge? Can I—and will I—fight for my life and win?

Thankfully, each of us in this book has won. Still, we feel sobered by the fact that far too many other gallant warriors in this endless war battled just as bravely, yet lost the fight. We cannot and will not forget them.

I wish our new friends you are about to meet could have coached me fourteen years ago on how to boost my immune system; on the enormous healing value of friendships and the importance of giving and accepting love; on how to get the facts by teaming up with doctors, therapists, and technicians; and above all, on the many ways to keep one's spirit energized and mind effectively set.

You will find some powerful principles here. These winners offer dozens of small tips and major truths that help us prevail not only over cancer, but over any other unwelcome event life throws at us. As you read, you'll also realize an inescapable truth about yourself: *You are an overcomer.* Overcomers maximize life. They persevere. They expect to prevail.

Each of these cancer survivors has generously offered his or her experience in the hope that it will help, inspire, and encourage you. That is the deepest desire of my own heart as well, and the reason this book was written.

INTRODUCTION

Information in this book is not intended to promote specific medical or cancer treatment centers, medical or other treatments, therapies, or cancer protocols. The reader should diligently seek the best in current medical knowledge and treatments, determine to participate fully in his or her chosen treatment course, and rejoice that the healing arts today include multiple effective approaches to successfully surviving cancer.

HOW TO USE THIS BOOK

Whether you are a cancer survivor, a cancer patient, or the friend or relative of either, you are now a member of an organization you never sought to join—an organization of people who have experienced the pain, emotions, and raw courage that this disease can bring forth.

Surviving Cancer is the inspirational product of one remarkable woman's victory over cancer, centered on seven basic principles that became her prescription for success.

This book is filled with stories and practical applications to help you understand and cope with what you or someone you love may experience during cancer treatment. On the following pages, graphic symbols are used to illustrate:

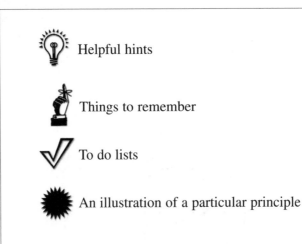

Helpful hints

Things to remember

To do lists

An illustration of a particular principle

There are also areas throughout the book for journalizing as well as detailed reviews of each of the seven principles at the end of certain chapters.

Think of *Surviving Cancer* as a workbook—a manual to get you through the most important project of your life. Keep this book handy, mark pages of special interest, scribble notes and inspirational thoughts throughout, refer to it often, and share it with friends and loved ones. *Surviving Cancer* delivers a strong dose of reality concerning the cancer treatment experience along with a message of hope from those who not only survived, but also thrived. Our best to you in *Surviving Cancer.*

CHAPTER 1

SURVIVING
CANCER

If cancer were to strike you or someone you love, would survival be the outcome? Millions of us have had to stare that loaded question in the face. The good news, according to the American Cancer Society's Year 2000 figures, is that some eight million Americans alive today have recovered from cancers of every type.[1] Important research, diagnostic, drug, and treatment breakthroughs are happening as this is written, with even more hopeful and highly promising news on the horizon.

But this book's primary mission is not to report on new weapons in the cancer war, but to examine the tremendous changes taking place within cancer patients themselves. Today's patient is far more proactive and involved with treatment options than ever before. He or she is far less willing to passively accept a cancer verdict. As knowledge about cancers becomes more readily available to the lay person, the medical community has come to expect patients' active involvement in fostering their own cure. Teamwork has become the norm and often results in spectacular success.

This book has been written by a breast cancer survivor who deeply desires the same wonderful outcome or one even better, for you and others. Like the thousands of other cancer patients and survivors I have interviewed during the past fifteen years, I simply wanted to know the best ways to help myself weather the most threatening health crisis of my life.

As thousands of other former cancer patients like me told what worked for them, these seven powerful survival principles emerged:

- Take charge
- Get all the facts
- Strive for optimum health
- Boost your immune defenses
- Love more
- Adopt faith, hope, and optimism
- Maximize life

Certain other fascinating traits seem nearly universal among those who once battled cancer. For example:

- If we entered our cancer battle as a wimp, we emerged as a fighter.

- We learned to take aggressive charge over our disease, treatments, and health, and appreciate the good health we were born with.

- Cancer caused us to examine our attitudes toward life and resolve to live more fully and generously.

- Our personal relationships became more important to us—more involved and honest.

- We changed our lifestyle in significant ways: everything from nutrition, exercise, and stress relief, to finding time for travel, learning, adventure, and fun.

- We feel lasting gratitude for life and its good gifts.

- We passionately desire to help and encourage others who may be dealing with cancer.

What Cancer Survivors Know

Believe it or not, many cancer survivors say they actually feel thankful for the challenge thrust upon them by their particular life-threatening disease. It stops you in your tracks. It makes you think—and re-think. Some people relate how cancer toughened them up as they tapped into their inner resources, while others say it makes them sensitive toward life, the people they love, and the beauty around them.

Most report that cancer taught them the vital importance of researching one's diagnosis, learning all one can about the specific disease, and entering into treatment partnerships with physicians one respects and deeply trusts.

Most report that cancer taught them the vital importance of researching one's diagnosis, learning all one can about the specific disease, and entering into treatment partnerships with physicians one respects and deeply trusts.

Others, however, relate regrets about not getting second medical opinions, listening to their own inner doubts, or taking time to study their options thoroughly and make informed medical decisions. Very often people say they acted in haste. A few people in this book say they wish they had done things differently, and honestly tell us why.

REMEMBER

A cancer survivor with good sense and a fighting spirit can do far more to encourage another cancer patient than any clinician who hasn't "been there."

Secret No More

More than one doctor has remarked that a cancer survivor with good sense and a fighting spirit can do far more to encourage another cancer patient than any clinician who hasn't "been there." I believe that's true, probably because I didn't have such input. Fifteen years ago, I believed that of all the people my husband, Glenn, and I knew, I was the only one with cancer. I wondered why I, a healthy, youthful, energetic woman, had been singled out.

Today, of course, I know that couldn't possibly have been true. Cancer strikes one in every three American families.[2] Every one of us, therefore, is somehow affected by cancer: our own, a family member's, or that of someone else we admire, love, or hold dear.

But nobody talked about cancer then—at least not often, and seldom publicly. If you had a mastectomy, your friends weren't likely to know. Even those few years ago, cancer still was the silent killer, the C-word was so dreaded that you felt reluctant to speak it aloud. But less than two decades later, America's attitudes toward cancer have swung dramatically away from silence, fear, and passive accept-ance—none of which is my style anyhow!

Today we fight. We form groups. We race for the cure. We inform ourselves via the internet and other means. Eager to tell others what we have learned through hard experience, we survivors march, telephone, E-mail, and speak before civic groups, television audiences, and even the U.S. Congress.

But it gets even more personal. How often a frightened voice on the telephone, usually someone I don't know, has resulted in my accompanying another woman to her oncolo-gist's office to support her, listen with her, and perhaps even ask questions she might not think to ask. Or perhaps it's a young husband and father, devastated by the news that his wife's cancer might take her from him and their children in less than six months. (In that case I suggested avenues they might explore. The young woman's "incurable" cancer, once widespread, has been in remission for more than five years.)

Yes, we survivors, once cured, often continue to fight. We raise money for cancer research and tell our govern-ment, loudly and insistently, that we must have more fund-ing, more research, and the national determination to stamp out cancer in our lifetime. Many doctors believe this could be achieved. Some say prostate cancer, for example, could be vanquished within the next decade.

My Cancer Story

I have names of more than one thousand cancer patients—many, possibly most, now survivors—in my Rolodex files.

HINT

America's attitudes toward cancer have swung dramatically away from silence, fear, and passive acceptance.

Usually their doctors referred these patients to me. Fifteen years ago, my cancer led me into intense study of nutrition and the benefits of nutritional supplementation. I spent hundreds of hours learning from some of the world's foremost experts on the subject, not only studying their published scientific reports, but often meeting them in face-to-face interviews they graciously granted. I read countless stacks of medical literature, avidly absorbing everything I could learn about nutrition and the human immune system. I believed my future depended upon this knowledge—and I was right about that.

Before cancer, as a highly successful businesswoman with widely publicized and lucrative fashion showrooms in New York and Dallas, I believed I was living the best possible life. Dee Simmons at forty-seven was a former beauty queen, a beloved wife, mother of a gorgeous and talented daughter, blessed with high energy, and—I thought—excellent health.

Then came breast cancer, mastectomy, and reconstructive surgery. I was blessed to have the finest medical treatment and a successful outcome. But the nagging question remained: Why had this cancer happened?

As I recuperated, a paper with an amazing story came into my hands. I read this cancer survivor's testimony about her cure through nutritional supplementation and was galvanized. Knowing almost nothing about nutrition, which at that time was largely ignored by the medical community, I immediately charged into a leading local health food store and began learning about vitamins, free radicals, the immune system, and a host of other topics I knew virtually nothing about.

Talk About It

Soon I became a convert, telling my cancer story on television and sharing my ever-growing knowledge about nutrition. Doctors, not trained in medical school about the subject, began referring patients to me for counseling they were not able to provide.

Glenn and I often speak of the amazing turn in the road my destiny took, and how radically our lives and personal commitments have changed as a result. My years since cancer have been packed with learning, interviewing, and studying. There have been many eighteen-hour days and countless late night telephone opportunities spent encouraging and informing cancer patients who call me from every part of the globe.

Ten years following my cancer experience, I established a business which distributes the nutritional and skin care products I had created originally for my own use, insisting that they be as pure, high-quality, and effective as can be devised. Glenn suggested that I name my company "Ultimate Living," because we were determined to aim for the highest and best living, not just the marginal health styles so many of us are content to accept.

Ultimate Living International, Inc., continues to research and create the most potent line of nutritional and wellness aids available anywhere. I insist on that. You might say I'm betting my life, at least to a significant degree, on it. And it is with true gratitude that we offer our line of immune-enhancing items to other cancer patients, survivors, and others who know the vital importance of undergirding their physical systems with the best in nutrition.

The point of all this, however, is to say that my present knowledge of nutrition, my widespread nutrition company, my hundreds of appearances on television programs, network shows, and speaker's platforms, all began with another woman's testimonial, printed at her local print shop and distributed as best she could.

Her story and ideas changed my life. It made me seriously consider nutrition, lifestyle, and wellness for the first time ever and put me somewhat ahead of the curve at that time in spreading some cancer-fighting news. I continue to spread the proactive wellness message, and so should you.

What We Tell Others

"What did you do?"

Cancer patients who want to hear my story always begin with that question. First, let me stress, I do not prescribe. Cancers and cancer patients differ widely from case to case, and of course I am not medically trained. However, I gladly offer facts and suggestions about how to research, locate the best physicians, and discover new approaches and treatment centers without ever urging anyone to take one path or another. Such decisions belong to the patient, and given enough facts, most of us are quite able to decide for ourselves.

But certain cancer survivors, I among them, have accumulated a considerable body of factual knowledge about the subject. I think of two prominent prostate cancer survivors. Dr. Richard Howe, retired president of the Pennzoil Company, and Michael Milken, the noted philanthropist, are described by top-level medical specialists as possessing a breadth of knowledge about prostate cancer, rivaling that of many practicing urologists and oncologists. Dedicated to learning everything possible about their disease, these brilliant lay authorities stay abreast of current scientific developments, foster the causes of prostate cancer support groups, and raise desperately needed funds for research.

2

Such decisions belong to the patient, and given enough facts, most of us are quite able to decide for ourselves.

Though Dick Howe and Mike Milken, operating separately and on their own initiative, freely supply their immense knowledge to the rest of us, they nevertheless are careful not to practice medicine.

Other Suggestions

In brief, here are some of the cancer-survivorship principles I pass along to others. These commonsense and well-tested suggestions work on several levels.

1. Take charge. Get all the facts you can about your cancer and how to fight it. Then lead your own parade. Make informed decisions, and form your own rules about how you plan to handle this challenge. It has been observed that proactive patients actually gain stronger immune defenses. Tell yourself, "I am in charge here."

2. Look on your healing journey not as a chore, but as a blessing. This may sound strange, even impossible, but those who adopt that approach seem to handle cancer treatments well. One patient had a strenuous multidisciplinary course of treatments for pancreatic cancer, a type nearly always incurable, which included surgery, radiation, and chemotherapy. Throughout several hospital stays and months of treatment, she remained emotionally sturdy, and she decided not to focus on the treatments or how she felt, but instead to use her time creatively. During her stays at the hospital and intermittent trips home, she regularly prayed for her doctors and other clinical staff. Now healthy, she has little memory of cancer as a dificult experience. She actually remembers it as a life-changing and wonderful time.

What Frieda Did

3. Gather your resources. Recently diagnosed with breast cancer, Frieda Courson of Atlanta immediately swung into action on her own behalf. At first dazed and somewhat disbelieving, as we all are when we get the news, Frieda and her husband, Tom, drew up their to-do list within a matter of hours.

The couple's lives center around their Christian faith, so prayer for wisdom, strength, and guidance was the first order of the day. Out came Frieda's address book from which she gleaned names of those who might help her: a fellow church member connected to the American Cancer Society, a friend who could use the internet, several others who had experienced breast cancer, and a medical journalist.

Frieda scheduled herself for the first available surgery slot at her local breast clinic and within days underwent a lumpectomy procedure. Meanwhile, she continued to telephone, study her options, and get details of her health insurance plan in place. Despite this non-stop activity, Frieda and Tom kept their spirits up by following, and praying over, the detailed action plan they had created.

The final task was that of choosing among three leading cancer centers known to friends who recommended them for their providing state-of-the-art medicine. After prayer, Frieda telephoned each of the three and chose a center world-renowned for success with curing breast cancers. Accepted immediately, she traveled to the out-of-state cancer resource center and was accepted into a clinical trial being conducted there, but instead of staying there, she returned to Atlanta and decided with her local oncologist on a similar protocol. She felt fully informed and comfortable with her decision.

Frieda Courson modeled a nearly seamless way of intelligently approaching what for many, if not most, seems a devastating personal challenge. She marshaled every bit of information and other resources she could find. She wasted no time, tackling the project immediately. She asked others to help with telephone calls, information gathering, references, and advice. The whole thing, from diagnosis, surgery, examination at the out-of-state cancer center, to beginning her nine and one-half month course of radiation and chemotherapy, took little more than one month—despite heavy medical and airline schedules during the late year holiday rush!

"We lined up our resources and did everything possible so we'd feel we had made the absolute finest medical decisions," Frieda says. "Tom and I went into this battle thoroughly prepared. I feel peace about the treatments and confident about the outcome."

That's the whole idea. Above all, gather your resources.

Cooperate and Change

- Take time to study.
- Make your game plan.
- Stick to it.

4. Get on the program and don't waver. Can you imagine that some people actually walk away from scheduled cancer treatments? Others accept treatments with resentment and generally disbelieve or argue with doctors' advice. This is not the time to vacillate. Instead, take time to study and make your game plan (see above), and then stick to it! Do your best to cooperate. Take an interest in your doctors and caregivers. Cooperate, stay the course, and do everything in your power to survive.

5. Change your lifestyle. I wondered why I, of all people, got cancer. But you should have seen the way I ate. I'd bake these to-die-for chocolate chip cookies (yes, maybe literally!), crammed with double chocolate and double nuts. I'd eat ten or so with my morning coffee—before breakfast! I could go on (it gets even worse), but you get the picture. I ate lots of food, anything and everything, stayed skinny, and never thought about nutrition.

Obviously, I knew I'd have to change my ways, and I have. I am far healthier today, in fact, than I was when cancer struck. But we have to stick with those changes life-long. We must plan to survive and keep on surviving—no more choosing doughnuts instead of vitamins.

Emotions and Stress

6. Talk about your emotions. Every time I talk with cancer patients, I ask about their emotional state during the two years prior to diagnosis. "Everything was fine, nothing wrong," most say, until later in the conversation they begin to recall a trauma or a long period of stress due to divorce, job loss, financial struggle, an abusive spouse, death of someone close to them, or a long list of other reasons.

It never fails. Even little children recall losing a pet, a friend, a grandmother, or experiencing the pain of their parents' divorce. We must find ways to acknowledge such pain, loss, stress, or failure in our lives, which can actually affect us at a cellular level.

Survivors realize that we absolutely must mend relationships, rid ourselves of undue stress, and make personal peace a priority. We need to actively set the emotional stage for survival. We should focus on expressing our emotions, positive or negative, and healing those that afflict us.

For me, that realization proved illuminating. I had a very happy life, a good marriage, and the world's best husband. My world seemed nearly perfect. Honest reflection, however, showed I had been ignoring some important and basic needs while I achieved the business success which seemed so satisfying.

At that time we were building an elaborate, costly house for our family. D'Andra, our beautiful teenager, was going through a stage of emotional turmoil. Add to that the incessant travel and long hours my fast-track business required, and it all spelled big-time stress. I now know that stress can kill. At that time, like most other Americans, I simply ignored it.

But we worked through the emotional and stress-building issues. The house got built, the daughter grew up, and both turned out beautifully. The real decision, however, was to close down my fashion showrooms and walk away from "my" scene. I never regretted the decision. Today I pay attention to stress factors and have learned to recognize and discharge emotional overloads immediately. This protects the immune system, which was designed to protect me, keeping me healthy and cancer-free.

Powerful Weapons

7. Cancer is the ultimate battle. I tell patients they must fight it with all they've got. Fight it with your mind, body, and spirit. Enlist others to fight alongside you: your husband or wife, your parents, pastor, boss, close friends, and all those people you don't think of at first who quietly show up and offer to help. Let them.

Also, don't underestimate your own abilities to rise to the challenge. We all have far more inner resources than we dream we have; now is the time to discover them and use them. We each came into this world with an amazing ability to surmount all sorts of obstacles and to heal. Far more than we can possibly imagine, we are built to heal.

Cancer is the ultimate battle. Fight it with your mind, body, and spirit.

8. Use your faith. Most people have religious faith to at least some degree, and most survivors tell at length some of the ways they called upon their faith during their cancer experience. We'll say more about that in a later chapter, but now it is important to acknowledge that countless medical studies, ongoing and completed, describe the major role religious belief plays in a patient's healing. Even if you have walked away from the faith you held earlier in your life, there's no better time to return to it.

Stories That Inspire

There are thousands of thrilling stories about those who have survived cancer—most filled with commonsense, practical attitudes, and advice. You learn a lot about human courage, too. As I was led to one story after another while writing this book, my motive was to set forth some of the survival principles that shine forth from them. These simple but vitally important principles can be easy to overlook or ignore. Also, I was fascinated to discover what other cancer survivors have learned from their life-threatening experiences.

These accounts came to me randomly. They were not chosen via any elaborate testing pattern, but were meant to display individual attitudes, courage, and brainpower at work.

I found plenty of all the above. These people mirror you and me: some old, some young, some ordinary working people, others wealthy and privileged, with every sort of cancer challenge in the book. Many once deemed incurable are alive, thriving, and immersed in great projects. They represent dynamic proof that there is life after cancer—in many cases, very abundant life.

But there's another fact I've seen again and again, and that is that there's some undeniable yet unidentifiable factor in survivors' personalities that even experienced clinicians can't seem to name or describe.

Survival Factor

What is that distinct survival factor? I cannot say. But as one nurse at a well-known cancer treatment facility admitted to me, "You can tell within minutes whether a patient, no matter how early or advanced the cancer may be, will live. I can't explain how, but you can tell." Doctors sometimes declare it a mystery as to why two patients with the same disease at the same stage and in the same general health will experience two completely different outcomes to medical treatment.

This is not a simple question, but one which all interested in medicine and healing must address. We survivors, interested in helping others to survive, find ourselves pondering: Why did I live? Why did she succumb? What makes the difference?

"You can tell within minutes whether a patient, no matter how early or advanced the cancer may be, will live. I can't explain how, but you can tell."

We don't pretend you will find the answers to such imponderable questions in this book. But you will find some underlying and well-tested principles that embrace not only surviving, but overcoming, prevailing, and resuming full-blown life with a capital "L."

Read on, and see what the human body and mind are capable of accomplishing. Imagine, too, the breadth and scope of the human spirit. We all know celebrity cancer survivors who have become a sort of folk hero, someone larger than life, but the fact is, you and I are made of the same material. If celebrities can be conquerors, we can be conquerors too.

A Second Chance

As Lance Armstrong, the cyclist who won the Tour de France after surviving cancer, has said, "Sometimes in life you are given a second chance. If you are given a second chance, go for it." The man Susan Wales and her daughter,

Megan Chrane, met in Atlanta one day must have had the same belief. Shopping in a busy mall for college items, Megan stopped short at a kiosk where she had spotted a "really cool" cellular telephone. As Susan reminded her daughter, somewhat heatedly, that they were shopping for necessities, not another gadget, a young man they had noticed standing nearby approached them.

"He looked very Hollywood," said Susan, an author, speaker, and executive producer who lives in Pacific Palisades. "There was the leather jacket, designer jeans, bleached hair. He really startled me."

It turned out that the young man had a purpose. He first introduced himself, then immediately explained that he was a cancer survivor and that he wanted to give Megan the phone she so obviously wanted. As Susan struggled to form an answer, he explained.

"I had malignant melanoma. I wasn't supposed to live. My dad owned a large chain of restaurants on the West Coast and we had plenty of money for the best treatment in the world, but you can't buy what I needed.

"I promised myself then that if I got well, I would try to make other people happy."

He turned to Megan, a firm expression on his face, and added, "I want to give you this telephone, but I have a condition. In return, I want you to promise me that you'll do acts of kindness for three different people."

5

"I want you to promise me that you'll do acts of kindness for three different people."

Megan, obviously touched by this unusual encounter, readily accepted. "She felt humbled by his story and his generosity," her mother related. "Megan has no problem with doing kind things for others, but perhaps she really needed to meet someone who was so very grateful for a second chance at life. Every time she uses that telephone, she'll stop and think."

Today those precious second chances at life arrive more and more frequently. People mentioned in this chapter and numerous others like them, all survivors, cherish life as few others in the population can imagine.

We had some tough battles to fight, but by the grace of God and relentless efforts on the part of our doctors and medical community, we managed to win. As so many of us can testify, the cancer experience, no matter how challenging, can transform us, our relationships, and our purpose. Ultimately, it can help reveal the true meaning of our life.

7

"Sometimes in life you are given a second chance. If you are given a second chance, go for it."

MY THOUGHTS

If I am given a second chance my life is defanetly going to change. I need less stress and more time and love for my kids & Don.

MY THOUGHTS

CHAPTER 2

THE CONTAGIOUS POWER OF HOPE

I call *hope* the world's most powerful medicine. Though science can't measure its effects, and no one can absolutely assess its power, most doctors can recall at least one "incurable" patient who, for unknown and unsuspected reasons, slid over into the winner's column. Often clinicians attribute such results to something intangible they call *hope*. Virtually everyone I have talked to, doctor and patient alike, spoke about the important role hope plays in achieving healing.

The tragic fact remains, however, that too many thousands of gallant patients fighting cancer hope, pray, work, endure, and believe, yet do not survive. The last thing I want this book to suggest is that those who lose to cancer despite their most intense and heroic efforts are somehow less capable than those who survive. I passionately resist that idea. I know that beating cancer requires far more than mere denial, some glib self-help prescription, or a philosophy of mind over matter.

Painfully, I think of those in my own extremely sturdy and unusually healthy family who have had to fight this war. My grandmother died of cancer, for example, yet I had breast cancer and survived. In 1989 we went through my beloved mother's battle with pancreatic cancer and her swift death from the disease. In this past year alone, our family again has been hit hard by my only sister's breast cancer, which she is successfully combating, and our eighty-two-year-old father's surprising diagnosis of prostate cancer. His tremendously elevated Prostate-Specific Antigen (psa) levels were discovered only months following a normal reading and revealed widespread involvement. He recently went to be with the Lord.

No wonder I hate cancer! And that's just one American family, a group of apparently healthy, vigorous movers and shakers, most faith-filled, none passive or prone to negative thinking. I am sure you can imagine, therefore, why for many years I have anguished and wondered, why? What makes the difference between survival and loss? And what can we do, really, to significantly increase our chances for survival?

Let's return to the seven principles most of our interviewees and medical authorities have continually stressed:

- Take charge of your case.
- Get all the facts. Inform yourself thoroughly.
- Eat only the foods that provide optimum nutrition.
- Boost your immune system.
- Express your feelings. Love helps you heal.
- Adopt faith, hope, and optimism.
- During and after cancer, resolve to live each day of your life to the fullest.

These principles work. Whether in sickness or in health, most of us could take our lives to a much higher level. But for the cancer patient in particular, according to hundreds of men, women, and doctors I talked to, these seven baseline principles might just make all the difference.

The decision to take our life and health more seriously, and to provide ourselves with every available physical, mental, and emotional benefit, provides us with countless reasons to hope. So let's do it. Let's hope for the best outcome. Hope for full recovery and a long life. Hope for a victory and for future prosperity. Now, that's really good medicine!

Potent Medicine

A legendary African-American musician gave a wonderful word-picture of hope when he described his feelings on leaving the hospital following prostate cancer surgery.

"The same raggedy street, Sunset Boulevard, I've been going down for thirty-five or forty years, all of a sudden looked like the Garden of Eden. The green in the trees was the most beautiful green I've ever seen in my life. People's eyes...I mean, I'd never seen these things before...."

That was one man's poetic description of the deep awakening many of us feel following initial surgery, chemotherapy, or tumor radiation treatment. No matter our pain, discomfort, or anxieties, here comes this sudden jolt of real, deep-down, core-of-our-being hope—hope so fierce and indescribable, compounded from amazement at being alive, experiencing aliveness in the "greenest greens" around us, and despite momentary pain or weakness, ardently willing ourselves to keep this awe alive within us.

It must have been that same instinct of hope which made one cancer survivor schedule her wedding between chemotherapy sessions following her breast cancer surgery.

The treatments, she said, felt like "you're being hit with a baseball bat." Nevertheless, she planned her wedding and elaborate reception at a time when, as she described herself, she was "bald as an egg" and felt relentlessly sick. The groom, exhausted from tending her, had contracted a viral infection and was running a 102-degree temperature.

Though that's certainly not the romantic wedding most girls dream of having, there's a happy ending. Now recovered from her strenuous cancer treatments and regaining more strength and vitality each day, she has returned to her busy career with her usual verve and zest. Her hair has returned too, and there's every prospect for a "proper honeymoon" when her work allows.

Life goes on, and hope makes so much of life become possible. This cancer survivor portrays the very essence of hope. It is a role any of us can play. *This, too, will pass. Things will get better. Of course we will survive this, and then comes the honeymoon.*

Like a golden thread of enormous tensile strength, you'll glimpse the attitude of hope weaving through so many of our winners' stories. Long after they recover, it still shines from their faces.

Power for Your Future

We cannot be whole, or fully healed, unless we are excited about our future. The woman mentioned above demonstrated that she fully intended to participate in her own happy future. And while few cancer patients actually hold their wedding while in the midst of arduous medical treatments, it's good medicine to plan *something* that will be important to us.

A co-ed who was being treated for lymphoma chose her chemotherapy sessions as a good time to thumb through catalogues and fashion magazines with her mother. Together they chose her college wardrobe as they ignored the chemo drip. Oddly enough, the girl never got sick from the treatments.

A man receiving radiation therapy for vocal cord cancer was ordered not to speak, or even to whisper, but since he was neither sick nor weak, he made a list of tasks he could

REMEMBER

The Seven Principles

- Take charge of your case.
- Get all the facts. Inform yourself thoroughly.
- Eat only the foods that provide optimum nutrition.
- Boost your immune system.
- Express your feelings. Love helps you heal.
- Adopt faith, hope, and optimism.
- During and after cancer, resolve to live each day of your life to the fullest.

Hope for the best outcome. Hope for full recovery and a long life. Hope for a victory and for future prosperity.

No matter our pain, discomfort, or anxieties, here comes this sudden jolt of real, deep-down, core-of-our-being hope.

tackle during his "silent season." One thing he did during those long weeks was to organize his extensive collection of musical scores, in preparation for the possibility that he later could resume singing. Now fully recovered, he sings as beautifully as before cancer. Does hope play a significant role in such success stories? Though there's no way to prove it, I strongly believe it does.

Sick or well, it's vitally important that we look forward, actively and positively, to tomorrow. Cancer treatments and recovery from surgeries sometimes can seem to take forever, especially to us impatient people, but we can occupy ourselves constructively during those months with making some great plans for the future. Otherwise, a state of hopelessness or, at the very least, a flat sort of boredom, will set in. That creates a climate in which serious physical, emotional, and spiritual problems can develop.

The staff of the famous Menninger Foundation, once asked to identify the single most important factor in treating the emotionally disturbed, unanimously declared hope to be of primary importance. They confessed they had no idea of how to infuse a patient with hope. It is an elusive gift. Nevertheless, they could immediately discern when a patient turned that crucial corner, because hope changes all of us for the better.

Hope helps us heal. It literally powers our future.

Researching the Role of Hope in Health

HINT

During treatment it's good medicine to plan *something* that will be important to you.

Martin E.P. Seligman, Ph.D., in 1991 published *Learned Optimism,* a much-discussed book that describes the effects of optimism and psychological therapy on health. He declares that studies convincingly show that hopelessness or pessimism depletes the immune system. In the years since then, other studies have shown the same evidence, which few clinicians today would dare to dispute.

Dr. Seligman and his research team embarked on work using cognitive therapy to boost the immune systems of forty patients then undergoing standard medical treatments for colon cancers and melanomas, with a control group using no mind-body therapies.

The study reported exciting increases in the numbers of natural killer cells among those patients receiving cognitive therapy (the deliberate changing of hopeless or pessimistic thinking), whereas there was no change in those patients in the control group. "In short, cognitive therapy strongly enhanced immune activity—just as we hoped it would," he wrote.[1]

REMEMBER

Sick or well, it's vitally important that we look forward, actively and positively, to tomorrow.

In his book entitled *Reinventing Medicine,* Larry Dossey, M.D., says there is evidence that "acting as if" can produce medically significant changes in the body, and that our actions can produce effects on the body that have important health consequences. "Acting as if" we are being

TO-DO

Occupy yourself constructively during those months of treatment and recovery with making some great plans for the future.

■

The staff of the famous Menninger Foundation identify the single most important factor in treating the emotionally disturbed as Hope.

■

healed or, in other words, actively practicing hope, according to Dossey, actually leaves tracks on the body.

He tells of researchers who studied the impact of people's optimism on their health. In half a dozen studies involving more than 51,000 men and women aged 19 to 94, the question asked was simple: "What do you think about your health?" Those groups included a broad spectrum of health conditions and such lifestyle factors as smoking cigarettes, yet all the studies showed the same conclusion: The best possible predictor of survival for the next decade is the answer people give to that question.

"Those who say their health is 'poor' are *seven* times more likely to die than those who say their health is 'excellent,'" Dr. Dossey wrote.[3]

Hope Is Contagious

Among the numbers of psycho-immunological studies, where hope seems universally agreed upon as a vitally important element in healing, one important aspect, it seems to me, is routinely omitted.

The *contagious* power of hope gets left out in those interesting scientifically measured studies in which patients answer questionnaires and have their immune responses measured via blood tests.

Such studies do not speak of the power of the patient's hope to raise hope in others: his or her family, other patients, and even one's doctors or other staff personnel. One patient with liver cancer, for example, told of how he enjoyed having nurses gather around his hospital bed "just to talk," and how interested he was in hearing about their lives and their concerns. His serene and confident spirit, his own unflagging hope, drew others to him like a magnet.

Contagious hope tends to spread quickly from one person to another, at home or in a hospital room. We should all intentionally spread this potent medicine to those around us.

REMEMBER

Hope helps us heal. It literally powers our future.

Hope Helps Us Make Plans

What motivates us to dig in our heels and battle through the toughest times in our lives? What helps us believe in our bodies and their ability to heal? What keeps us excited about the future?

Destinae Rae, an Evergreen, Colorado mother of five, a singer, and, incidentally, a cancer survivor, illustrates the motivating power of hope. The tall, auburn-haired songbird was just thirty-eight when she discovered a lump in her breast—too young, her doctor believed, to suspect cancer.

The doctor was terribly wrong. When I interviewed Destinae on *Health Views,* my health-oriented television program, she spoke of her cancer treatments. Today, following fourteen surgeries and two courses of chemo and radiation therapies, the vibrant, beautiful, and still youthful Destinae described some of the mindsets that pointed her toward ultimate healing.

"Acting as if" can produce medically significant changes in the body.

First, of course, she credits God, the doctors, and other therapists whose skills led her into extraordinary success with healing, breast reconstruction, and survival. But I was even more intrigued by Destinae's attitude of faith and enthusiasm about her future during those long months of treatments.

Destinae Rae exudes hope and personal power. I asked her where that energy and strength come from. What kept her so excited about her future? Why, during her lowest physical ebb, did she make such daring plans for her future?

Destinae's brown eyes sparkled as she answered my questions. "My strength comes from God, of course," she quickly replied. "But there was a skiing accident when I was fifteen..."

HINT

"Those who say their health is 'poor' are *seven* times more likely to die than those who say their health is 'excellent.'"

It was a bad one. The teenager suffered massive head injuries in that near-fatal mishap. "My parents started praying," she recounted. "The doctors were amazed that I lived, that I needed no brain surgeries, and that I had no facial destruction."

Amazingly, the pretty teen survived the terrifying ski accident without sustaining permanent cosmetic damage. The person within, however, had been changed forever. During that crucial and tenuous time, Destinae dedicated her young life to God. She says that decision created in her a strong determination to survive, which carried over years later, into her eventual cancer fight. Those God-given survival instincts, she believes, strongly guided her feelings about her future.

"From age fifteen, I believed there was some kind of ministry ahead for me," she related. "I wanted to discover what ministry. Of course, I also wanted to see my children grow up. And beyond that, I had a burning desire to launch my singing career."

Quite simply, Destinae Rae had no intention of allowing cancer to derail her life and her goals. For one thing, she wanted to record her songs. She visualized fulfilling all her personal dreams, and, above all, continuing to mother her children and enjoy their developing lives. That was a tall order for someone undergoing the treatments Destinae Rae received, yet she never wavered. She kept her eyes on the prize.

6

Contagious hope tends to spread quickly from one person to another, at home or in a hospital room.

No matter how discouraging her circumstances might have seemed, Destinae never allowed hope to move away. It stayed just ahead, like the bright star that seems to precede us as we walk through a very dark night. Even after enduring a mastectomy, chemotherapy, and radiation sessions, then confirming that the small lump under her arm the doctor dismissed as scar tissue actually was, as she suspected, a return of her cancer, Destinae did not falter.

Her decisions and choices will be described later, but at this point we'll focus on how she maintained such enduring hope. "I did not doubt that I would live," she told me. "Never. There were my children; I had to live for them. I also believed I had a great future ahead, a future filled with my personal dreams. No matter how sick I got, I kept planning the albums I wanted to produce. I selected the songs, chose the program, even mentally designed my album covers."

However, choosing a photograph for the album at first gave her a reason for hesitation. Destinae had been told that chemotherapy powerful enough to destroy her cancer would also destroy her thick auburn hair. "I finally decided I'd just have to be photographed bald," she told me.

Things didn't work out that way. One morning Destinae took her children to a nearby McDonald's for breakfast, and a gentleman in the restaurant happened to compliment her on her long, coppery hair. "Thank you, but I may lose it soon," she murmured.

Moments later, the man approached their table and introduced himself. "My wife and I are missionaries," he explained. "When I told her what you said about your hair, she wondered if you might like me to pray with you."

Destinae and her children gladly accepted. "He prayed that my cancer would be completely cured. Then he prayed that I would not lose my hair," Destinae reported. Incredibly, despite receiving chemo's biggest guns and repeated courses of treatments, the stranger's prayer was answered. "I wish I could tell him my hair never did drop out," she says. "They told me the drugs I took *always* make that happen."

Hope reminds us of all we have survived thus far, of the sometimes terrifying challenges we have surmounted, and helps us to realize that we can survive new challenges

TO-DO

- **Make vivid plans for a fantastic life.**
- **Act as if you are perfectly healthy.**
- **Spread hope to others. Use it lavishly.**
- **Never, never, never forget to take your Vitamin H— hope.**

equally well. Hope also reminds us of all we have been given and all that we cherish. Hope tells us, again and again, that life is good. Hope instructs us to live our present and plan our future. Hope helps us focus, as Destinae did, not on what we fear losing, but on all we have to gain.

It is impossible to estimate the extent to which the habit of fostering hope, for our own selves or for a cancer patient, can affect one's eventual success. However, I can state one vitally important instruction about hope: *Never leave home without it.* Destinae Rae, and trainloads of others like her, will back me up on that.

MY THOUGHTS

Never give up hope. live oc try to live every. day to the fullest. Just knowing what ever the out come is I gave it all I had and never gave up hope I would be cured by God.

Principle 1
Take Charge!

What's the first thing you should do once cancer strikes? Take charge! Exercise your authority to establish your own guidelines as you tackle issues surrounding treatment options and a host of other personal decisions.

Be proactive, never passive. Choose how and where you will receive treatments. Select a team (spouse, parents, siblings, friends, coworkers) to advise and assist with daily needs. Also, most importantly, decide how you will nourish and bolster yourself throughout the treatment process. Attack your disease aggressively, make your own decisions, and fight to win.

Result: Taking charge produces a sense of control and helps us realize we are not victims, but overcomers. Anxieties are more easily banished, and feelings of confidence and well-being ensue. Deciding "I am in charge" enhances physical, mental, and emotional health.

TAKING CHARGE

"The news was like a rock falling on me," Dr. Richard C. Howe said, referring to his prostate cancer diagnosis.

One cancer survivor, informed that she had breast cancer, said the words simply did not penetrate. "It was like hearing words through a thick glass wall," she recalled. "I don't know if I was afraid or not."

And after another woman's breast cancer was diagnosed, she said she felt profound shock. "I wanted to believe it was untrue," she recalled. "Your body is failing you and has a disease, and it's not easy to accept." You may eat right, exercise, stay healthy and trim, have no family cancer history, and still learn you have cancer. The news hits everyone differently, but it always hits. Hard. In my own case, I remember feeling neither fear nor desperation because I shifted my problem onto Glenn, my loving and very protective husband. I avoided the issue emotionally by allowing him to take charge, and he did—willingly, intelligently, and thoroughly. Glenn always does things by the book, then goes even beyond the book. He searches every remote corner for correct information and best current advice.

And that's exactly what you must do, according to dozens of cancer survivors we interviewed. And, they unanimously agree, you need to get proactive about your case—immediately. Not everyone has a Glenn Simmons to meticulously gather information and informed advice. But even if you do, you'll soon learn, as I did, that it's my job to take charge over my body and its state of wellness and health. You can help and encourage me; encouragement is very welcome. But ultimately, my healing and future good health must become my own responsibility.

Becoming Proactive

Activity always strengthens us. That's especially true when we learn we have a cancer fight on our hands. Gathering information, making decisions, questioning former cancer patients, researching on the internet, all help place normal anxieties in perspective. We are doing something to help alleviate a condition over which at first we may feel temporarily powerless—an unfamiliar and unwelcome assault on our body.

If you are a list-maker, the time to begin is about thirty minutes after the diagnosis, or as soon as you pick yourself up. Most of us remember exactly where we were when we heard the news and what we did next. Perhaps we called a loved one or best friend, returned to the office without saying a word to anyone, drank a cappuccino or something stronger, or simply went home and cried. Immediately after the initial shock, however, the best thing we can do is to make a list of those who will help us.

On paper, write the names of your spouse, parents, children, pastor or rabbi, best friend, neighbors, coworkers, and siblings. Writing those names will warm and energize you. Those are the important others who will help you soldier through, the ones you can count on as you fight and win your battles.

You may be like one woman who at first could not bring herself to talk to anyone about her breast cancer. In fact, the then forty-four-year-old wife and mother of three told of leaving breast cancer articles around the house for her family to find because she couldn't bring herself to talk about it to her husband.

Treatment Options

Here's where we must bring all of our best intelligence and decision-making to the table. After one's cancer is diagnosed, it is important to search for the most knowledgeable specialists, surgeons, radiologists, and others available. These key choices can be arrived at by several means: your primary physician's recommendations, experiences of others treated by your doctor in the past, names offered by other clinicians in the field or gleaned from articles in medical journals or the internet.

Cream rises to the top, and as you and your friends persist in information-gathering, certain names probably will surface several times. It's a good idea to make appointments with at least two or three physicians noted for specializing in treating your particular cancer. At least two and ideally three separate diagnoses help solidify one's thinking.

"But my insurance plan doesn't pay for second opinions," some people object. "Get them anyhow," I always answer. "The hundred dollars you spend can buy priceless information, confirmation, and peace of mind." It's not uncommon for doctors to disagree about a diagnosis or treatment plan. If you receive two varying opinions, obviously a third physician should be consulted.

One woman's experience illustrates the advisability of getting multiple medical opinions. Her first doctor said she needed an immediate double mastectomy. The second said a single mastectomy, as soon as possible. Then someone in a large New York breast and ovarian cancer survivors' group suggested three leading oncologists she might contact.

"I called the first on the list at Memorial Sloan Kettering, a very upbeat guy," she said. "After he examined me, he said, 'I think we have a shot at a lumpectomy.'" The patient accepted that option, far less radical than those the other doctors proposed, with courses of chemotherapy and radiation following the surgery.

In all, she consulted three mainstream physicians and two or three alternative medical specialists before choosing the third doctor to direct her treatment protocol.

Tom Redmond of Minneapolis and Scottsdale, a retired CEO of an international hair care products company, also opted for three medical opinions when he learned he had prostate cancer. "Never stop at just one opinion," he warns. "The more you know about your illness, the better. Go to two or three specialists and let them advise you of your options. Friends and other cancer survivors also help. Doctors don't always help with the trauma. They are too clinical. But every man knows a friend who has gone through it before him. That friend can give invaluable help and advice."

Take Enough Time

Once cancer is discovered, we naturally want to attack the problem immediately. Treatment must be our first priority, of course, but only after we explore all possible options.

Take a man I'll call Hal, who received a lung cancer diagnosis and told his doctor, "Tell me what to do. I'll do whatever you say."

"Surgery. Tomorrow," his doctor replied. The operation was scheduled for the next morning. Hal's wife, meanwhile, began investigating cancer treatment centers that

HINT

If you are a list-maker, the time to begin is about thirty minutes after the diagnosis, or as soon as you pick yourself up.

TO-DO

On paper, write the names of your spouse, parents, children, pastor or rabbi, best friend, neighbors, co-workers, and siblings.

specialized in lung cancer. When his niece, a nurse, telephoned from a famous clinic offering Uncle Hal the possibility of entering a clinical trial there, he demurred.

"I promised my doctor he could operate first thing tomorrow morning," he said. Unwilling to wait long enough to get even one more opinion, Hal passed up the opportunity to receive state-of-the-art treatment for his illness. Possibly even that might not have helped, but Hal's outcome was not good, and his widow still regrets their not pursuing other possible options.

Another woman related that when her mammogram showed a tumor that proved malignant and her doctor advised a mastectomy, her first impulse was to agree. But a chance encounter with a woman who had survived breast cancer with her breast intact led her to seek a second opinion. A few weeks later she had a less invasive lumpectomy and has recovered well.

After one's cancer is diagnosed, it is important to search for the most knowledgeable specialists, surgeons, radiologists, and others available.

As most cancer survivors learn, sometimes regrettably after the fact, it is rarely necessary to make a quick decision about treatment. It is far more important to learn what your options are and discover—before you do anything else—all you possibly can about the disease. No one ever regrets taking those steps.

"When three doctors give you the same diagnosis and recommendations about treatment, you face whatever surgery and medical treatments you need with confidence," Tom Redmond explained. "Take your time. Get all the facts possible before you proceed."

Ask the Right Questions

I can't count all the times I have accompanied someone else to an oncologist's office for a review of his or her cancer case. It is always a good idea to have a second pair of ears, incidentally, to make sure you understand the information and ask the questions you need answered. But if you don't care to have someone else along or have no one to ask, I suggest bringing along a small tape recorder or, at least, a notepad and pen to record the doctor's observations.

Here are some questions you need to ask:

- What is the proper name of the cancer I have?

    Ask your doctor to spell it, if necessary.

- What stage is it?

- Will I need surgery? What kind? When?

- Has the cancer spread, or is it in situ?

- What other treatments will I need?

By the time you have compared answered to these questions from two or three separate physicians, confidence in your ability to make excellent choices and decision should be firmly in place.

Changing Doctors

Sometimes even a good doctor's best advice does not resonate with one's gut feelings about the illness. Perhaps he or she comes across as too clinical, brusque, or intimidating. Whatever the situation, the two of you seem not

HINT

It's a good idea to make appointments with at least two or three physicians noted for specializing in treating your particular cancer.

REMEMBER

If you receive two varying opinions, obviously a third physician should be consulted.

emotionally or personally in sync. At times like these, several interviewees warned, it's wise to leave—*immediately*.

Does it pay at such times to trust your instincts? I believe it does. You may have a long, hard fight ahead, possibly even a life-or-death struggle. It only makes sense to put together the best medical team you can find, those with whom you feel not only confident, but also comfortable. It's great when your attending physician is someone you really like, as well as trust.

"Never stop at just one opinion. The more you know about your illness, the better."

A man who survived cancer of the larynx described the compassionate attitude his oncologist at New York's Memorial Sloan Kettering hospital displayed. "Smoking tobacco and consuming alcohol causes the kind of cancer you have," the doctor informed him. Then he added gently, "But we didn't know that in the past. Don't blame yourself. You didn't know." His words eased the patient's heart. Later the doctor's expertise saved not only the man's life, but also his voice.

By contrast, a well-known television journalist told of approaching her breast cancer with a reporter's thorough list of questions for her surgeon. When he became annoyed, she left and found another surgeon to perform her bilateral mastectomy. "Don't pat me on the head and tell me, 'That's okay, dear. I know best,'" the journalist concluded. Her attitude, according to many cancer specialists, was perfect. Get the facts. Insist on teamwork.

Back in the days when you signed a consent form, were anesthetized, and awoke from surgery to discover whether or not you still had a breast, another woman I know said her surgeon told her, "Just sign here. You are forty-one and divorced. Losing a useless appendage isn't going to matter all that much. You can still lead a normal, productive life."

She didn't sign. She found another surgeon who excised the lump and found it innocent. Before she departed from the city's leading oncologist, however, she advised him, "If you lost only a little toe, you could still live a normal, productive life. However, I'd hope you'd ask a few questions before you signed a consent paper!"

Sometimes, Tom Redmond would agree, it really pays to choose your doctor not only with your head, but also with your heart. You deserve not only the best medical treatment available, but also a physician who practices common sense, caring, and compassion. For those rare, unsatisfactory doctor-patient relationships, cancer survivors offer a strong word of advice: *Leave!*

REMEMBER

It is rarely necessary to make a quick decision about treatment. It is far more important to learn what your options are and discover— before you do anything else— all you possibly can about the disease.

Choosing a Treatment Center

As cancer research progresses and treatments and cure rates improve, treatment centers dedicated solely to cancer patients' care and cure continue to proliferate. The newest of these can supply not only a full range of state-of-the-art surgery and other medical treatments, but many adjunctive aids as well—nutrition classes, relaxation, arts and crafts, faith-based resources, and beauty shops with aestheticians who teach patients how to look and feel their best.

REMEMBER

It is always a good idea to have a second pair of ears, incidentally, to make sure you understand the information and ask the questions you need answered.

TO-DO

Bring along a small tape recorder or, at least, a notepad and pen to record the doctor's observations.

Individuals we interviewed who received cancer treatments at such centers were enthusiastic about the concept of treating not just the cancer, but the whole person. Destinae Rae, who entered the Cancer Treatment Centers of America, located in Tulsa, Oklahoma, during her second bout of breast cancer, found the experience very different from the more conventional path she took the first time.

Destinae says being encouraged to bring her faith to the forefront increased her confidence and reinforced her determination to participate fully in her healing process. She cites the careful use of standard medical procedures combined with equal emphasis on rebuilding the immune system by nutrition and other means.

"The idea is to treat the individual, not just the cancer," she explained, adding that she believes the approach resulted in far less damage to healthy cells than other modalities might do.

Second-time cancer treatments can be strenuous, but Destinae downplays the idea. "What I remember is riding a bicycle during one hundred degree summer heat!" she teases. Now recovered, healthy and strong, Destinae Rae helps others plan cancer fact-finding and information-gathering needs. Like most other recovered cancer patients, she is quick to encourage others to battle for their cure and believes strongly in a holistic approach to the cancer challenges.

Treatment centers like the one Destinae entered are located in many large cities. Even more numerous, however, are the better-known and even famous hospitals and clinics devoted not only to cancer treatments, but to cancer research as well. Here varieties of clinical trials test new drugs and techniques, and varieties of modalities can be combined to treat individual needs. Some of the facilities offer the best medical hope the world can provide, and patients mingle with others from many other parts of the globe.

How, then, do you choose a treatment facility that is best for you? One way to begin, some suggest, is to seek hospitals in the forefront of research for your type of cancer. Two examples: (1) Houston's M.D. Anderson has a broad spectrum of cancer expertise but is especially famed in the realm of prostate and breast cancer. (2) Dallas's U.T. Southwestern Medical Center has a world-renowned breast cancer center under the leadership of my friend, Dr. George Peters. Similarly, various hospitals and clinics lead the way in treating and curing specific cancers—melanoma, pancreatic, or prostate, for example—and it is not difficult to find which of these facilities might best serve you. Participation in clinical trials or access to state-of-the-art treatments might make the search well worthwhile.

Your doctor may know of new advances that could help you. The American Cancer Society can provide invaluable information. And from the internet you may discover interesting studies and new developments presently underway, and names of outstanding facilities and clinicians you might contact.

REMEMBER

Sometimes even a good doctor's best advice does not resonate with one's gut feelings about the illness. At times like these, several interviewees warned, it's wise to leave—*immediately.*

It makes sense to put together the best medical team you can find, those with whom you feel not only confident, but also comfortable.

REMEMBER

Get the facts. Insist on teamwork.

Difficult Cases

Most of us know all too little about cancers in general and our own cancer in particular. And should our case prove difficult or even be termed incurable, we hardly know where to start, much less how to take charge.

Now is the time to enlist everyone you know, from your physician to your mailman, to help you find ways to beat the verdict.

HINT

For those rare, unsatisfactory doctor-patient relationships, cancer survivors offer a strong word of advice: *Leave!*

Often this can be done. New treatments may save a limb or an eye or a life. Several of the cancer survivors discussed in this book had been called incurable yet today are living healthy, happy, and productive lives. New answers come along all the time, but it's up to us to find them.

The key to often miraculous success is persistence. Never give up. Keep looking for answers. Encourage others to help you search as well, because you never know when and how you may find the solution to your problem.

A man I'll call Jim is a perfect example of how help can arrive virtually at the last moment. At age eighty, Jim learned that an ordinary skin cancer on his forehead had spread to the underside of his eyelid. After surgery and several consultations with top specialists, all agreed that radiation would eradicate the cancer but destroy the healthy eye.

Jim, his wife, family, and friends swung into action, contacting doctors and clinics everywhere. Though the first priority was to rid Jim of the cancer, of course, his wife could not help believing there must be some way to heal the cancer and also save the eye. For several weeks, no answer appeared. Then just nine days before the scheduled surgery, one telephone call made the difference.

Surgery was canceled. Jim checked into another leading cancer treatment center and several weeks later returned home to recuperate. After a then new radiation therapy that pinpointed the cancer and spared good cells from excessive damage, Jim retained not only his healthy eye, but also a surprising amount of vision. Recently a final checkup revealed no trace of cancer or radiation damage, and the patient was told he is considered healed.

Such success stories come along far more often than we may realize. However, the path to success may not necessarily appear smooth. It may take countless phone calls and hours of seeking before you find the information you need, but even exhaustive efforts seem worthwhile when a cure is accomplished. And if it should turn out that I or a loved one did not receive a cure, I'd nevertheless want to know that I had made every effort.

No Place Like Home

While I believe in seeking everywhere for a successful outcome to one's cancer challenge, traveling to a distant facility is not necessarily the answer. More and more local hospitals and clinics provide excellent cancer treatments. Consultations with world famous specialists can be obtained via the internet. Sometimes delicate surgeries are directed from a distance via computer. Many, if not most,

I do not advocate leaving home to find good cancer treatments and care. I do advise, however, continuing to search for the best answer for your case and going to all lengths to find it.

■

✓

TO-DO

Follow the steps as you:

- Seek a diagnosis.
- Obtain second and third opinions.
- Choose specialists to treat your case.
- Research via several means.
- Choose where you will be treated.
- Learn everything you can about your illness.

■

open-and-shut cancer cases today are successfully treated and cured in hometowns everywhere.

When we learned I had breast cancer, my husband, Glenn, declared he'd take me to the best specialists anywhere in the world. After all his intensive research, however, the best place for me turned out to be at home in Dallas, with my care managed by Dr. Jim Peters, where I received superb medical care plus ample amounts of love and support from family and friends.

No, I do not advocate leaving home to find good cancer treatments and care. I do advise, however, continuing to search for the best answer for your case and going to all lengths to find it. This is perhaps the most important thing we can do to obtain a satisfactory outcome. As the Bible teaches, "Ask and keep on asking. Seek and keep on seeking. Knock and keep on knocking." (Luke 11:9.)

Take charge. Believe you can and will find answers for your needs. And above all, make yourself competent to decide how you want to handle your illness, your treatments, and your interim lifestyle. Those who actively approach these challenges say they believe those with confident, creative, and fighting spirits are most apt to win.

And as one man told me, "If I could beat this thing, you can too." Believe that, and go for it.

Principle 2
Get All the Facts

Learn absolutely everything you can about your cancer. Remember, knowledge is power.

Cancer survivors often sought second and third medical diagnoses and, in some cases, as many laboratory tests before deciding among treatment options. Get definitive answers about your cancer, they advise. What is the clinical name of the cancer? What stage is it? Will surgery be required? What other treatments will be needed?

Then comes some real research from the internet, medical specialists, medical libraries, and patients who have survived the same cancer. Record all such advice in a special notebook for future reference.

Result: Research at the outset often can save not only time and money, but, in some cases, life itself. Learning every possible fact about your cancer boosts your confidence in your medical team and your own decision-making abilities.

MY THOUGHTS

CHAPTER 4

PRACTICAL STRATEGIES

"**O**ur family never gave up. We worked really well together," one cancer winner told me. We all have options. No matter how tough things become, we have the option to figure out ways to prevail. People need a sense of control in order to feel good about life, and the first thing to remember is that you don't have to surrender normal controls. Cancer need not create chaos.

Strategizing and teamwork spell success in this situation, former cancer patients emphasize. They say this is no time to go it alone. To quote Charlie Brown, the beloved Peanuts comic character, "I need all the friends I can get."

Your Team

I've heard wonderful stories of how husbands and wives came through for ailing spouses during long, sometimes uncertain months of medical treatments. For me, my husband, Glenn, was my first and strongest line of defense. But you'll probably be surprised at how many others in your life step up and offer to help. Your gracious acceptance accomplishes two things: it lightens your load when you need it most, and it enables concerned relatives, friends, and co-workers to ease whatever apprehensions they may feel about your welfare.

A woman who says cancer made her physically weak for the first time in her life told of her hang-ups about accepting offers of help from others. At last, she chuckled, a crusty old family friend set her straight. "Your receiver is broke," he growled. "He was right," she admitted. "I learned a big lesson that day."

That's only one of many valuable life lessons a cancer experience can teach us. Other useful new ways of thinking and acting probably will occur, including the privilege and necessity of broadening our friendship circle as we allow formerly peripheral people to move closer to the center of our lives. "He was a neighbor I hardly knew, an older man," one man recalled. "When he learned I had melanoma, he rang the doorbell, said he had survived the same thing and wanted to encourage me. He coached me through surgery and chemo, and now I'm coaching him on the golf course." For some, the luxury of leaning back for a time and depending to some degree on the kindness of others is a needed, eye-opening experience.

False pride simply has no place in the cancer equation. There is something very beautiful and humbling about receiving the loving ministries of others—especially for those of us for whom giving seems natural, while receiving is sometimes hard. Hours after my own surgery, feeling exhausted, ill, and in pain, my friend Marian Barnes stood beside my bed and rubbed my cold feet in an attempt to love and comfort me. Years later, I still remember the warmth of her hands and the feel of her touch through those old bed socks they make you wear. I remember vividly her expression of love through that simple act of kindness.

Get accustomed to the concept of receiving from others. Realize that you'll need advice, ideas, and practical help from others, and occasionally you may even need to ask for aid. You may have to delegate some of your responsibilities to others for a time. Such unaccustomed shifts in this way of doing things can really bother an independent person, but we should remember two important truths:

1. Mankind was not designed to live and operate alone.

2. This, too, will pass. Relax and treat your serious but temporary cancer bout as just that—temporary.

Accepting such ideas is the initial step in gathering a good cancer-fighting team to accompany us into battle. Husband or wife, boyfriend or girlfriend, sons and daughters, your lawyer or fishing buddy, anyone you trust and

REMEMBER

False pride simply has no place in the cancer equation. There is something very beautiful and humbling about receiving the loving ministries of others.

HINT

Get accustomed to the concept of receiving from others. Realize that you'll need advice, ideas, and practical help from others, and occasionally you may even need to ask for aid.

REMEMBER

1. Mankind was not designed to live and operate alone.
2. This, too, will pass. Relax and treat your serious but temporary cancer bout as just that—temporary.

whose thinking you respect no doubt will volunteer for your squadron at the outset. Accept the gestures with thanks.

Problem Solving

"I underwent surgery for breast cancer; the prognosis is for total recovery. I do not anticipate missing any oral arguments." The 1988 announcement from Sandra Day O'Connor, the first female justice of the U.S. Supreme Court, stunned the public. However, just five days after leaving the hospital, Justice O'Connor returned to the bench and was able to work despite receiving chemotherapy treatments.

Most of us want to handle our responsibilities as usual, and very often we can. We don't know how Sandra Day O'Connor managed her cancer treatments and the immense duties that concern the U.S. Supreme Court, but she is among many other U.S. Senators, corporate CEOs, schoolteachers, athletes, and others who somehow find it possible to carry on during treatments despite heavy schedules.

Each person's answer to such challenges is different, but all require individual adaptability and a knack for problem solving. For women, especially those who juggle job and household responsibilities, taking a cancer sabbatical, at first glance, might seem impossible. And for a male business owner who hasn't stopped to take a vacation in five years, apparently there's just no way. But in circumstances like those, winners bring their best planning skills to bear.

HINT

Most of us want to handle our responsibilities as usual, and very often we can.

As one man says, "When the going gets tough, the tough somehow, someway, will find solutions."

One path to solutions is to list, in special order, all the things that concern you. Include everything you need to do. Concerns may range from pet care to hair loss, from financial needs to worries about radiation therapy. Write it all down. The very act of writing siphons off a lot of anxiety. Then, separate your concerns into various categories: business, personal, medical, household, and so on.

The next step is to talk things over with those close to you. "We are all great communicators," one man remarked. Be direct and open as you express your fears, hopes, and needs. This proactive and very honest step strengthens family relationships enormously, as we learn, and in some amazing ways, solves some of the most bothersome problems.

"I worried about my dog. My daughter offered to take him until I finished my treatments. She knew he was spoiled, used to lots of attention, and wouldn't do well in a kennel. After that got solved, I didn't worry about a thing."

"I told my boss exactly what we might be looking at. He mentioned several options: unused sick leave and vacation time, working half time for a while, even working part time from home. As it turned out, I didn't have to miss much time at all."

"My nephew offered to do my yard work, my weekly grocery shopping, and drive me to clinic appointments. He

TO-DO

List, in special order, all the things that concern you. Include everything you need to do.

Then, separate your concerns into various categories: business, personal, medical, household, and so on.

Talk things over with those close to you.

Be direct and open as you express your fears, hopes, and needs.

Open up. Share your needs and anxieties with a certain few who will surely prove willing and eager to brainstorm with you.

■

TO-DO

Check with your insurance agent, your HMO manager, and the human resources director at work. Inform yourself about available benefits, and then estimate amounts of additional funds you may need. Consult with your spouse, accountant, banker, credit union, and others.

■

HINT

Such transactions as property mortgages should be handled early in the process.

■

helped me tremendously. When I asked what I could do for him, he said, 'Pass it on.'"

People are good. Most sincerely want to help, and benefits go both ways. While we want to keep life as normal and routine as possible, now is the time to relax those routines a little. So open up. Share your needs and anxieties with a certain few who will surely prove willing and eager to brainstorm with you. The following topics often arise.

Financial Matters

Check with your insurance agent, your HMO manager, and the human resources director at work. Inform yourself about available benefits, and then estimate amounts of additional funds you may need. Consult with your spouse, accountant, banker, credit union, and others who can suggest ways to obtain needed financial resources or remind you of assets you might otherwise overlook.

Example: People often don't think about borrowing against insurance policies or selling their second car. Explore your financial options.

Such transactions as property mortgages should be handled early in the process. And if you have decided to receive treatments in another city, you'll need to factor in future travel and lodging costs, as well as any medical tests and procedures not covered by your insurance plan. Should costs seem unmanageable, hospital officials sometimes are willing to work out long-term payment arrangements.

With a little research, you'll discover ways to keep travel and lodging costs within bounds. Some airlines provide special fare rates to cancer patients traveling to receive treatments. Many corporations provide free compassionate travel for patients and family members, allowing them to "piggyback" on corporate aircraft bound for business meetings in the appropriate city.

Hospital social workers usually can advise you of ways to cut travel and lodging costs. They can recommend nearby economical hotels, bed and breakfast inns, and special houses established to meet patients' needs. Most offer special patient rates plus such perks as kitchen privileges, free breakfasts, and shuttle service to and from hospitals and clinics.

Good Food

Nutrition becomes super-important at the very time some patients don't care much about eating. Hospitals, Caring Houses, and hotels' adjoining treatment facilities know this and make special efforts to tempt us to eat often and well. Strategically placed snack stations invite waiting-room occupants to maintain their fluid intake, and hospital volunteers continually offer fruit juices or soda.

By contrast, at home meals often can present a problem. Finicky patients become somewhat demanding or turn away from food. Even worse, the patient may be the one who ordinarily prepares the family's food and now has lost all interest.

HINT

Some airlines provide special fare rates to cancer patients traveling to receive treatments. Many corporations provide free compassionate travel for patients and family members, allowing them to "piggyback" on corporate aircraft bound for business meetings in the appropriate city.

HINT

It's the patient's job to decide to nourish him- or herself properly and to keep this discipline in place.
Solution: Designate a resident meal preparer or arrange to have good meals sent in.

REMEMBER

Meals on Wheels provides home cooking not just to the poor and elderly, but to anyone who needs nourishing hot food.

HINT

"Don't be so macho you insist on driving yourself to and from radiation or chemotherapy treatments." While some patients may take treatments easily in stride, others react differently.

Prepare for such possibilities in advance. It's the patient's job to decide to nourish him- or herself properly and to keep this discipline in place. Others must settle on how best to handle meal logistics and who will carry out such responsibilities.

This is extremely important and largely the patient's responsibility. I must promise myself that I will faithfully pursue a course of excellent nutrition, especially at a time when it contributes so much towards my physical and emotional well being and my ultimate cure.

Solution: Designate a resident meal preparer or arrange to have good meals sent in. Neighbors may offer to take turns preparing dinners. Even your young children, given a little help, may surprise you with their ability to produce decent meals. Remember, too, that Meals on Wheels provides home cooking not just to the poor and elderly, but to anyone who needs nourishing hot food. Costs are minimal, and the service is reliable and welcome.

Several cancer survivors we talked to advise certain transportation cautions. "Don't be so macho you insist on driving yourself to and from radiation or chemotherapy treatments," they advise. While some patients may take treatments easily in stride, others react differently. Plan to use OPT (Other People's Transportation) as offered or needed. Some treatment centers have special vans to transport patients to and from clinic appointments. Senior citizen centers may also offer medical transport for a reasonable fee.

Plan Your Work

"But what about my job responsibilities?" That burning question can cause great anxiety for some patients. The desire and need to work doesn't vanish because of one's changed personal circumstances. Indeed, work can provide much-needed balance to life during a cancer episode.

But how much should you confide in your superiors and colleagues? What do you tell them, and when? How can you realistically predict how much your illness will affect your work, and how long it may take you to recover?

Here's where talking things over with your spouse and friends really helps. Just airing some of these unanswerable questions helps clear your thinking and shakes everything down to reasonable bottom-line answers. These suggestions from other former cancer patients might start your thinking.

- Be honest. Tell your boss, partner, or team the facts, briefly.

- Keep a positive attitude—no fearful or hangdog expressions.

- Be ready to make suggestions about how to accomplish your normal workload.

- Approach work-related problems or challenges early, and ask others for suggestions. Do not feel threatened if someone else solves one of your thorniest work problems better than you might have done.

TO-DO

- Be honest. Tell your boss, partner, or team the facts, briefly.
- Keep a positive attitude—no fearful or hangdog expressions.
- Be ready to make suggestions about how to accomplish your normal workload.
- Approach work-related problems or challenges early, and ask others for suggestions. Do not feel threatened if someone else solves one of your thorniest work problems better than you might have done.
- Be as businesslike and professional as possible. Your attitudes will continue to rub off on those around you.
- Don't fear losing your job because you have cancer.

- Be as businesslike and professional as possible. Your attitudes will continue to rub off on those around you.

- Don't fear losing your job because you have cancer.

One man, who didn't want his name mentioned, experienced just that. When he informed his boss of his health status, he received sympathy and condolences and a pink slip. Irate, the newly diagnosed cancer patient sent out resumes far and wide, resulting in several job interviews. He was offered and accepted a high profile position in another city and began a "thrilling" new career while receiving cancer treatment. Once recovered, he rapidly climbed the corporate career ladder.

"Losing my job because of my cancer was the best thing that ever happened to me," he declares. "Of course, I was honest about it during future interviews, but nobody discriminated against me because of it. I'm sure such discrimination still happens, but it is out-of-step thinking. Temporary job adjustments can always be made."

- Don't expect more of yourself than you realistically can handle. Within realistic parameters, you can still do plenty of good work.

- Keep your sense of humor in the workplace. Not only will it help others lighten up, but it will also keep things in perspective for you.

- One businessman suggests approaching your business manager like this: "I was diagnosed with _____.

I will have (surgery, radiation, chemotherapy) in two weeks. I expect to be okay. I'd like to show Joe and Mary how I handle _____ so they can fill in for me, if need be. Meanwhile, I'll have time to finish the _____ project before my surgery."

The fact is, close relationships at home and on the job can keep you calm and help boost your immune system. And if at times you need to work from home, use technology to help you stay in touch with work issues. Both E-mail and the telephone can keep you connected.

You'll discover that plenty of other people have made such adjustments in their work lives. Ask how they coped. You have stores of creativity within you, and now is the time to bring it out. As you decide how you'll handle problems, large and small, details will fall in place and your confidence will increase.

Setting Boundaries

Think carefully about your time, energy, and commitments. Successful cancer patients neither underestimate nor overestimate these three factors. Ask yourself these two questions:

1. What really matters?

2. Do I have a hard time delegating?

By solving these two challenges of prioritizing and delegating, you may revolutionize your life. Most of us do far too many extraneous things, and cancer actually can help

Close relationships at home and on the job can keep you calm and help boost your immune system.

∎

REMEMBER

Think carefully about your time, energy, and commitments. Ask yourself these two questions:
1. What really matters?
2. Do I have a hard time delegating?

∎

TO-DO

Plan ahead.
Settle all
maintenance
issues as early
as possible—the
lawn, the leaky
faucet, the
scheduled
termite
inspection.

■

TO-DO

Sleepovers for
the kids,
grocery, dry-
cleaning, and
other deliveries,
housekeeping
services, and
the like, can all
be scheduled.

■

simplify, refresh, and stimulate our lives. The act of learning to delegate, as any harried and overworked individual knows, can give anyone's life a brilliant makeover.

Look forward to life. Plan the office party or neighborhood barbecue you'll host once this thing is over. Show others how much you appreciate them and how grateful you are for their friendship and caring.

Your Household

Plan ahead. Settle all maintenance issues as early as possible—the lawn, the leaky faucet, the scheduled termite inspection. "Get your car thoroughly checked and serviced right away," one fellow cracked. "Your wife may not do it."

Jokes aside, there's much you can plan at the outset of treatment that will make things run smoothly as time goes on. Sleepovers for the kids, grocery, dry-cleaning, and other deliveries, housekeeping services, and the like, can all be scheduled.

Telephoning takes time and energy. Assign as many of these duties as possible to others. Checking those mundane items off your list boosts your sense of control and peace of mind.

Beyond that, find a quiet, comfortable place you can call your own. A terrace, sunroom, or bedroom fitted with music, television, books, cushions, and anything else that adds to your feelings of pleasure and comfort contributes immeasurably to your recuperation and happiness. Feather your nest (or nests), and look forward to using and enjoying them.

To sum it all up, focus on the things you can control. List the activities in which you can make a difference. Learn how to say no. Fix your broken receiver. Confide in someone. And if it begins to dawn on you for the first time that you are far more important than your job, the tasks you do, or your role in life, your outlook will be transformed. Others can assume all the jobs you do, after all, but you—YOU!—remain priceless, unique, and irreplaceable.

Perhaps John Gray, Ph.D. and best-selling author, said it best: "Assume that everything will be okay—and relax."[1] That's a great prescription for life. I am one of the many cancer survivors who can testify that my experience taught me precisely that, and so much more.

In fact, everything is far more than okay. Life seems to get better, fuller, and more satisfying with each year that passes. Plan not just to survive, but to really live!

HINT

Find a quiet, comfortable place you can call your own. A terrace, sunroom, or bedroom fitted with music, television, books, cushions, and anything else that adds to your feelings of pleasure and comfort contributes immeasurably to your recuperation and happiness. Feather your nest (or nests), and look forward to using and enjoying them.

■

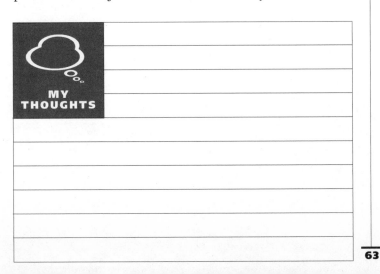

MY THOUGHTS

MY THOUGHTS

CHAPTER 5

THE BRAINPOWER PRINCIPLE

Several cancer survivors included in this book have headed large international corporations. Others also have earned considerable professional success. But every person quoted here, whether housewife or actress, home-builder or financial guru, holds one vitally important trait in common. Each recognized the power his or her brain exerts over the outcome of every effort we make. They understand how to use their brainpower.

Once we learn we have cancer, it's important to imme-diately tap into our mental resources to figure out how we'll handle our specific challenges. "I knew we needed to beat the odds," said a man during a television interview. "I had a bad diagnosis and a poor prognosis, which at first knocked me flat."

HINT

"I wrote a list of all the things I had going for me, and my wife added things I overlooked."

Then he put his mind to work. "I wrote a list of all the things I had going for me," he said. "My wife added things I overlooked. We agreed we were going to maximize every good thing in our life. If I did not survive, at least we'd have a happy ending.

"But we planned for me to live. We respected the doctors, but they don't always know everything. We decided to make a road map for how we wanted our present life—and our future—to go."

We all need a road map. It is exciting, even awesome, to see what our brain can propose and how faithfully our mind, body, and emotions can follow through. When our brain musters all our defenses, powerful results can occur.

Mind Power

We know the brain is the computer that manages and directs the body's every activity and movement. Boot up that computer and expect it to produce correct thinking, attitudes, and decisions. This will engender the confidence and steadfast peace of mind we all need during a crisis or serious challenge.

For many of us, cancer produced some valuable revelations. Because of cancer, I realized a simple, basic, and profound truth about my own lifestyle. I was a food junkie who absolutely disregarded certain laws of nature. I had never stopped to think, for example, that cookies, doughnuts, pies, candy bars, and so on, devoured regularly, whenever I wanted them, did not represent good nutrition. I was slender, energetic, and supposedly healthy, so a quick burst of energy from a big, sugary doughnut always seemed like a good idea.

Then came the day when the light bulb turned on. If I was going to attain good health and stay healthy, and if I was going to do everything I could to prevent future cancers and other diseases, I'd better switch on my mental computer and begin to learn how to change my ways. Like millions of other Americans, I was a healthy yet badly undernourished individual.

That one thought, that personal decision, marked a huge turning point in my life, my husband's health, our marriage, and my future career. Had I not experienced cancer, I might have continued to waltz through life with a typical mediocre health pattern and eventual lowered energy and stamina, and perhaps even a shortened life span.

As any cancer survivor knows, your thinking changes in several ways as you take on the challenge of saving your life. But what so many of us don't realize at first is the crucial importance of using that powerful brain to set our course, determine our attitudes, and protect us from detrimental beliefs, feelings, and decisions.

"Garbage in, garbage out," according to computer gurus. Now is the time to put good stuff in and give no space to negative thoughts and feelings. This may not seem easy, but it is essential.

HINT

Now is the time to put good stuff in and give no space to negative thoughts and feelings.

You Are Still You

The first information your mental computer should program is the fact that you are still you. My "take charge" message (I say those words repeatedly as I counsel and encourage hundreds of cancer patients) means, among other things, that you should keep your life going the way you want it to go. Your personality, beliefs, and little individual quirks and habits are still in place, and the successful way you usually run your life will determine how successfully you handle a really serious personal circumstance—cancer.

Put your own stamp on things. Think of ways you can avoid the pale-patient-lying-in-bed syndrome. Think of ways to surmount the real and debilitating illness. I'm thinking of teenage Sabrina, battling Stage Four Hodgkin's disease, who took an orange to peel and sniff during her chemotherapy sessions. Focusing on the fruit's rich color and sharp citrus scent helped offset any tendency toward nausea.

That was Sabrina's own prescription, and it worked. Doctors would no doubt call the girl's homemade solution to nausea the placebo effect—a phenomenon in which someone believes a particular neutral substance will make them feel better. It is that strong belief, the mind's power, which effects the relief. Scientists believe our natural internal painkillers, endorphins, under the mind's direction act to bring us relief from pain, nausea, and other discomforts.

Think about ways to enhance your comfort and offset possible unwanted effects of illness, medications, and treatments.

HINT

Put your own stamp on things. Think of ways you can avoid the pale-patient- lying-in-bed syndrome.

You know yourself better than anyone else does. With thought, we can all direct and control far more about our situations than we may realize at first.

Connie experimented with ways to control nausea caused by her strenuous treatments. She decided always to eat a simple, easily digested breakfast a couple of hours before chemotherapy treatments. Whether because of her mindset, her own reasoned approach to the problem, or the food itself, it usually worked.

She also had a back-up precaution in case it didn't, however. She kept a toothbrush and toothpaste with her at all times. "I didn't think about getting sick, but if I did, I'd immediately brush my teeth and rinse my mouth, and I'd feel fine. I didn't think about nausea or dread it, and it seldom happened. When it did, I didn't dwell on sick feelings."

More than twenty years ago an Atlanta teenager with advanced Hodgkin's disease underwent extensive radiation therapy which always resulted in vomiting. (Radiation therapy has advanced greatly since then, of course, so there's little reason to expect ill effects.) Melissa and a friend agreed to pray each morning, five minutes ahead of her treatments, believing all would go well and Melissa would experience no nausea.

From the first day, the plan worked. "She begged me to take her out to lunch that day," her mother recalled. "She wanted a chili dog, fries, and chocolate milk. That sounded like a bad idea to me, but she said, 'Mom, we prayed!' That meal might have made an adult sick, but my daughter ate every bite and enjoyed it."

That orange, toothbrush, and prayer, all simple, individual answers to a common and unpleasant problem, show the power of the mind. Cancer teaches us many ways to tap into that power and find innovative solutions.

Your solutions might differ from mine, Connie's, Sabrina's, or Melissa's. You, after all, are not just another cancer patient. You are you, and you can find your own successful solutions.

Time To Think

TO-DO

Set aside a specific time each day to think.

That's when you clear your mind and think through the day's activities and decide how you will handle things.

There's a lot going on in our lives as we fight cancer. There are multiple decisions to make, detours to take, and practical problems to iron out in addition to conquering the disease itself. "It's a full-time job," one man grumped.

That's why it makes sense to set aside a specific time each day to think. If you habitually pray, meditate, or read inspirational materials at a certain time each day, "thinking time" could also be included.

That's when you clear your mind and think through the day's activities and decide how you will handle things. That's when you'll get the inspiration to take along an orange, for example, or remind yourself to ask a medical question you keep forgetting.

Thinking time centers us. It gives us a strong approach to the day. It helps us keep problems in perspective, ask needed questions, and above all, think beyond ourselves into the lives of others we love.

Schedule time to think. Now, more than ever, it matters.

Expectations

"How much will this hurt?" That's a good question but always hard to quantify since pain is subjective. Your surgeon can offer some idea of pain usually associated with a particular procedure. So can others who have experienced it. Still, you are you. Your experience will be entirely your own, not related to anyone else's.

Why do we differ so widely in our susceptibility to pain? I once thought some people are naturally more sensitive than others. We have all heard the expression "high (or low) threshold of pain."

But what about self-fulfilling prophecies? If I expect something to be painful, won't my mind tell me I should hurt? I believe in thorough information-gathering regarding any treatments I expect to receive, including information from friends who have already experienced the same procedure. But their perceptions of pain, nausea, weakness, or other discomforts need not make me expect identical effects in my own case.

Example: Strong perfumes give my friend headaches. The scent of strong perfume does not affect me in the same way. However, if I expected perfume to bring on a headache, as it does with my friend, I'm sure a headache would appear.

REMEMBER

Positive
expectations go
a long way
toward
improving not
only one's
outlook, but
also the actual
situation.

- If other
  women can
  handle this,
  I can too.
- I intend to
  handle my
  treatments
  well.
- If I expect
  to become
  weak, I will
  feel weak. I
  will use my
  strength and
  become even
  stronger.
- I heal rapidly.
- After surgery,
  I want to get
  out of bed
  and walk as
  soon as
  possible.
- I'm not up to
  my usual
  exercise
  schedule, but
  I can
  accomplish
  plenty by
  walking or
  biking ten
  minutes at a
  time, three
  or four times
  a day.

I have learned first to prepare myself with appropriate information, and then to keep an open mind. I need not predict or expect negative effects. Should they appear, I'll know what to do. But I need not choose to think or imagine various side effects into existence.

Positive expectations go a long way toward improving not only one's outlook, but also the actual situation. Here are some examples of the kind of thinking and self-talk our winners used:

- If other women can handle this, I can too.
- I intend to handle my treatments well.
- If I expect to become weak, I will feel weak. I will use my strength and become even stronger.
- I heal rapidly.
- After surgery, I want to get out of bed and walk as soon as possible.
- I'm not up to my usual exercise schedule, but I can accomplish plenty by walking or biking ten minutes at a time, three or four times a day.

But it's not just intending, or saying such things, that makes them happen. We have to discipline ourselves to believe, really believe, that it is possible to achieve the good results we tell ourselves we need and desire.

Mental Pictures

The late Dr. Norman Vincent Peale, noted minister, author, and speaker, believed the images that affect us most strongly are self images. The author of the bestselling book *The Power of Positive Thinking* wrote and lectured extensively on the dynamic role the brain plays in guiding our actions and lives. Imaging, particularly self-imaging, holds an enormous influence over how we succeed in managing our lives, Dr. Peale believed.[1]

Sophisticated people at first discounted the positive thinking thesis. For years other ministers and therapists scorned the idea as simplistic and naïve. During the half-century since Peale's book was published, however, science has learned much more about the brain. Scientific and popular thinking on the subject has evolved to the point where most of us today know we can pattern our thinking, alter our self-image, and radically change our lives. Indeed, most cancer centers teach patients to monitor their self-talk and think positively.

Those individuals who say they are healthy have considerably longer life spans than those who believe themselves to be in poor health.

At any point in life, it's a good idea to administer a self-test regarding our self-image. But anyone who faces a major health challenge should make a point of doing so. A man who often mentors other businesspeople advises anyone facing personal challenges to list in writing all the assets that are working in one's favor.

Example: I am physically fit; my wife supports me in every possible way; we have good insurance; my kids love me, etc.

Those individuals who say they are healthy have considerably longer life spans than those who believe themselves to be in poor health.

■

TO-DO

A man who often mentors other businesspeople advises anyone facing personal challenges to list in writing all the assets that are working in one's favor.

■

REMEMBER

Your brain is an incredibly creative tool. Learn to use it to direct your images of yourself as someone incredibly capable of acquiring the health, strength, and healing you desire.

TO-DO

When you list everything—and it may take several pages—you hold in your hands an excellent, up-to-date self-portrait.

REMEMBER

Remember, no one deserves cancer—least of all, you. Picture yourself as vibrantly healthy, brimming with energy, effectiveness, and an overflowing appreciation for life.

When you list everything—and it may take several pages—you hold in your hands an excellent, up-to-date self-portrait. It is amazing how making that list can change your self-concept and help positive mental images replace weak or uncertain ones.

Form the discipline of creating strong mental images about yourself, your family, your work, your friends, and your medical team. Use your thinking time to picture strong results and good outcomes.

Your brain is an incredibly creative tool. Learn to use it to direct your images of yourself as someone incredibly capable of acquiring the health, strength, and healing you desire. This is not hocus-pocus, but proven good science. Plenty of studies show the importance of having a healthy self-image. In sickness or in health, we can control the picture of ourselves that we keep in our mind. We can strengthen and improve that picture day by day, indefinitely.

Above all else, believe you deserve healing and good health. Remember, no one deserves cancer—least of all, you. Picture yourself as vibrantly healthy, brimming with energy, effectiveness, and an overflowing appreciation for life. You can have all that, and more.

Desire and Healing

Couple your strongest emotions with the awesome power of your brain, and you can give serious illness a double whammy. Right thinking, a healthy imagination, and an ardent desire for healing and health make a potent combination.

Tom Redmond has described his self-prescription for helping him keep his prostate cancer at bay. "I ride my horses, enjoy nature's beauty, and appreciate my life," he said. So many other cancer survivors express similar sentiments. The initial desire simply to live seems to intensify and expand once the crisis is passed, and universal human instincts toward beauty, truth, and savoring life's goodness translate into new, deep desires to experience life more fully.

Perhaps that desire in itself represents a healing from the disease of too much busyness–the rush, fatigue, and staleness so many people call "life."

Think of the cancer survivors you know, and you realize how wise, effective, and content they seem compared to others in the general population. Few seem bitter or angry; most are glad and grateful. And if you smoke, don't ask a cancer survivor for a cigarette, because he or she won't have one!

The strong desire for a healthy lifestyle, which emerged during my own cancer experience, is still hard to describe. Perhaps some deep-seated life force powered my hunger to learn the facts about wellness that I needed to know. I desired the kind of health and vitality I had begun to envision. That desire fueled my lifestyle from then on, with results past all I could ever imagine!

Think of the cancer survivors you know, and you realize how wise, effective, and content they seem compared to others in the general population.

Fifteen years ago this then forty-seven-year-old, recuperating cancer patient, still weak and in pain, began to desire healing and full health. That desire was to create phenomenal change and radical new growth in my person, my marriage, and my life's mission.

Get in touch with your deepest desires, and I promise you'll receive benefits you've never dreamed you could attain. Visualize your desires. Speak your desires aloud and write them on paper. Practice picturing the deep desires of your heart. Consciously keep them before you, and your brain will do the rest.

As Dr. Peale said, "Prayerize, visualize, and actualize."[2] It works.

Brain Energy

To plot any intelligent course of belief or action, we need brain energy. It makes sense, then, to set aside needed quiet time so brain "juices" can flow. Scattered energies, emotions, and activities drain the mental energy we need for successful thoughts and healing.

Many recovered cancer patients echo these beliefs. Several mentioned the importance of feeding one's self positive, reinforcing thoughts at bedtime. This practice leads to better sleep and soaks the subconscious with good ideas and hopeful feelings.

One certain brain energy booster is to remind yourself, regularly and habitually, that if others can achieve good health, so can you. No matter how ill or weak a person may be, repeating the fact that we indeed are entitled to possess good health, signals the brain to carry out the process.

To activate brain energy, to get all mental cylinders firing, remind yourself of a few cogent facts:

- The mind needs definite instructions. Example: I am eating three full meals and two healthy snacks today.

- Monitor what you think and what you say to others. Example: I plan to take a photography course next fall.

- Focus on where you want to go, not on where you are at present. Example: Next week I'll begin to walk again. I'll start by walking around the block.

- Create celebrations and rewards for yourself and your friends. Host a bedside pizza party. Order a book or an audio album, or plan a movie night at home.

- Each day plan to do something "normal." At times such small tasks as feeding the dog, brushing your child's hair, or writing a note to a friend feel like major victories. Go for it! Send your brain the message, "We're moving right along!"

- Each day build in some fun wherever possible. Laughter, most agree, is still the best medicine.

The Discipline of Optimism

Some people are born optimists, and others must learn how to become optimistic. If this mind-boosting trait does not come naturally, remember that it can be learned. How?

By training yourself to deliberately focus on the positive—and believe. Throughout the day, every day, remind yourself that you are okay and things are getting better.

Here are some of the ways survivors learn to transcend their negative feelings by focusing on the positive:

- Remind yourself that we are winning the cancer war. Cancers are being detected and treated earlier, and more people are being healed.

- Treatments are improving, with increasing effectiveness coupled with fewer unpleasant side effects.

- The elderly can handle strenuous cancer treatment regimens as well as the more youthful. They have as much right to expect successful cures as anyone else.

- While certain drugs cause hair thinning or loss, others do not affect hair follicles. Your doctor can tell you what to expect, so you can plan accordingly. Any hair loss will be temporary. It nearly always grows back.

- Fatigue and weakness may happen, but not always. So you have a few quiet days. Is that a bad thing? Expect to stay strong, however, and your body may well obey your brain's commands.

How much are you willing to expect and believe that the best is really up to you? And when you discipline yourself to do just that, give yourself a priceless bonus.

Use your mind to expect the absolute best every day of your life. Learn to look at the benefits or adversity—and there *are* always benefits. Begin to plan for a wonderful future. Each day think about specific pleasures you will enjoy in the months ahead.

There's no time like the present, cancer patients say, to plan a garden, a vacation, or the future decorating job on the living room. One woman, a widow, used her long months of treatment and recuperation to study investing for the first time in her life. Thanks to diligent study and some good luck, she eventually tripled her investment income. "Before cancer, I never had the opportunity to learn about finance," she explained. "I was always too busy."

Seeing *opportunities* instead of limitations leads us into the healthiest, most prosperous form of optimism. Even while fighting cancer, you truly can enjoy time for introspection; time to know your family better; time to form new business plans; and time to read valuable, mind-expanding books or listen to every recording of your favorite artist or composer.

Use your brain. Pursue only the highest and the best. Picture only the beautiful. Imagine only happy occurrences. Remember only the greatest days of your life. Look forward to perfect success and radiant good health.

That is optimism, my friend, the kind that so often works healing marvels. And now, here are two stories of women who took an optimistic approach to their inevitable chemo-induced hair loss. The first, Jennifer, decided she'd seize the opportunity to completely change her persona. "Only total baldness and a wide range of fabulous wigs could offer the opportunity," she deadpanned.

HINT

There's no time like the present, cancer patients say, to plan a garden, a vacation, or the future decorating job on the living room.

∎

Seeing *opportunities* instead of limitations leads us into the healthiest, most prosperous form of optimism.

∎

Jennifer went shopping. She bought wigs that suited her various personalities, she explained. There was the wild, curly, Little Orphan Annie look; the sultry brunette, Cleopatra look; and the glamorous blonde. Friends never knew whom Jen might choose to be on any given day, but she always played the role and had fun doing it. "I never knew if that black-haired wig turned me into Dragon Lady, or if I chose it because I was Dragon Lady that day," she remarked.

Most of us, however, react more like Mary Elaine, who shopped for wigs and found exactly what she wanted—a hair color, texture, and style so close to her natural hair that only her closest friends knew she was wearing one. "I *insisted,*" she reminded me. "I would accept nothing less than total deception." Then came the day when Mary Elaine discovered her ruse would no longer work. "Treatments were over and my hair was growing back—fast," she said. "One morning I realized, however, that my wig was now passe. My new hair was not only thicker and curlier than the hair I lost, but was as blonde as it was when I was in high school."

What does an optimist do in a situation like that? "I tossed the old wig, the old style, the old color, and went with my new short 'do,'" she said. "I also bought new earrings, not serious ones like the ones I usually wore, but big gold hoops, some dangling stars, and some toucans. My hair is looking really good, but my earrings get all the attention."

They say we actually use only five or ten percent of our available brain capacity. Put another five percent or so into fighting cancer, your own or someone else's, into living the life of an optimist, and great things can happen.

Guide your destiny now as never before. Think how best to control the events of your life, to make yourself happier, and to treat yourself well. Cancer may not turn you into a curly-haired natural blonde, but it can teach us to use our brainpower for a successful, optimistic present and a triumphant, healthy future.

MY THOUGHTS

MY THOUGHTS

CHAPTER ❻

FOOD THAT BUILDS GREAT HEALTH

Talk to any cancer survivor, and you're likely to find someone who has become passionate about the role diet plays in overcoming illness and attaining excellent health.

Michael Milken's research on the subject made him believe so strongly in the importance of low-fat, nutritious foods, including soy and other ingredients, in fighting cancer and heart disease that he developed two healthy foods cookbooks.* Destinae Rae, once her cancer was diagnosed, went straight to a nutritionist for advice about the best diet and dietary supplements for her critical needs.

And while recuperating from breast cancer surgery, I plunged into the study of nutrition, at that time not yet a mainstream topic, and ended up devising for myself a mixture of natural supplements to fight any cancer cells in my body. Those potent supplements, rich in fiber and crammed with natural enzymes, minerals, amino acids, vitamins, antioxidants, and natural whole foods visibly improved my health and boosted my energy amazingly.

That was a case of "find a need and fill it." I intended to enhance my immune system as much as possible. Obviously it needed help, I reasoned, or I would not have contracted cancer. So, with advice from some of the world's leading nutritionists and scientists, I chose my ingredients and combined them to my own specifications. I wanted organic and the purest, most carefully chosen combination of all natural ingredients for my purpose—that of restoring and saving my life.

Does that sound too dramatic? I didn't think so at the time, and still don't today. After all, a large part of your body's construction and successful operation depends on your lifetime food consumption. "You are what you eat" may be an old, trite expression, but my favorite guinea pig—myself—has thrived on my recent, cancer-inspired dedication to nutrition.

There's nothing like a cancer experience to make you sit up and take notice of what you're putting into your body.

There's nothing like a cancer experience to make you sit up and take notice of what you're putting into your body. No more junk food for me, I decided at the time. My body needed help *right now*. The mixture I whipped up in my kitchen provided just that.

Today we know mixtures like the one I concocted for myself as "nutriceuticals." Such natural foods, produced to pharmaceutical standards, actually prevent disease or even may stop illness in its tracks. While knowledge about cancer-fighting foods is fairly commonplace today, such rapidly accumulating information has been gathered mainly in the past decade or so.

The American Cancer Society says that one-third of all cancers could be prevented by dietary means alone.[1] They advocate eating five to nine servings of fruits and vegetables, plus whole grain foods, daily. That sounds simple enough. Our prosperous society certainly makes the right foods available to most of us, but *we don't eat them.* The cost of our fast-food lifestyle and unbalanced eating habits has become enormous. But as people like me will tell you, old, careless eating styles come to a screeching halt once we learn we have cancer.

Making that 180-degree dietary turn, for me, meant intensely studying nutrition, consulting many of the world's leading researchers in the field, and, closer to home, buying a juicer and pouring good stuff into my body. For Dee Simmons, no more junk. I really meant business.

As it turned out, I did mean business. Eventually the concoction I had mixed for myself would become distributed worldwide. I named it Green Miracle, because the life-giving green foods packed into the all-natural powder seemed to work miracles for me and for others. This was the first nutriceutical I devised. It became the flagship product of Ultimate Living International, Inc., the company I formed to distribute Green Miracle and other super-pure and potent diet supplements and skin care products.

The Basics

But I'm getting ahead of myself. Like many other supposedly healthy individuals who suddenly find themselves confronted by cancer, I was amazingly ignorant about the true importance of the foods we eat. Glenn and I considered ourselves discerning diners. We are accustomed to enjoying exquisite meals in some of the world's finest restaurants. But as even some of the wealthiest baby boomers are discovering, you can habitually dine like a king yet suffer woeful malnutrition.

If we consume enough of the right foods, we can confidently expect to ward off most cancers.

We must return to basic good nutrition. If we consume enough of the right foods, we can confidently expect to ward off most cancers. Develop sloppy dietary habits, however, and we pay the price in obesity, heart disease, diabetes, cancer, and other serious illnesses. Glenn and I still enjoy gourmet dining, right down to an occasional sinful dessert, but we always first make sure our daily basic food needs are met. Our Green Miracle, for example, provides the daily equivalent of a pound-and-a-half of fruits and vegetables.

Nationwide, the word is spreading about the benefits of diet in cancer and other disease prevention. The American Cancer Society and other authoritative health sources continually urge us to adopt a nutrition plan consistent with the 1992 U.S. Department of Agriculture (USDA) Food Guide

Pyramid, the 1995 Dietary Guidelines for Americans, and similar recommendations from other agencies for preventing a host of diet-related chronic illnesses.

In brief, the food pyramid is built on a broad foundation of grains, fruits, vegetables, and nuts, with meat, poultry, fish, and dairy products assigned a smaller role. Eating as few as five to seven servings of fruits and veggies per day has been shown to offer effective defense against free radicals in the body which cause cancer. A serving is considered one-half cup, far less than the average restaurant salad.

Eating as few as five to seven servings of fruits and veggies per day has been shown to offer effective defense against free radicals in the body which cause cancer.

A pilot study at the AMC Cancer Research Center in Lakewood, Colorado, had twenty-eight women aged twenty-eight to eighty, all at risk for breast cancer, eat ten or more daily servings of a diverse group of vegetables and fruits for just two weeks. At that point, blood samples were taken which showed DNA damage to their white blood cells had dropped 21.5 percent—in just fourteen days![2]

Think you can't possibly eat nine or ten servings of fruits and veggies per day? You might be surprised. A tall glass of orange, grape, or cranberry juice counts as two servings. A yummy dessert of strawberries not only tastes fabulous, but helps fight cancer. You can get two servings of fruit in a delicious smoothie made with low-fat milk, strawberries, and bananas.

Another good way to boost cancer prevention is simply with whole grain breads. Eat brown rice instead of white, oatmeal instead of wimpier breakfast cereals. I enjoy the extra flavor whole grains give to foods.

As for protein, you can't beat fatty fish such as salmon for Omega 3 benefits to the heart and protection at the cellular level.

Take time to browse the supermarket with a whole new agenda in mind. Personally, I shop the outer edge of a market since I purchase only fresh food.

Fight Cancer Even at a Picnic

Deliberately choose cancer-fighting foods whenever you eat anything at all—yes, even on a picnic: mini-pizzas made with whole wheat English muffins, tomato sauce, chicken, olives, and cheese; chunks of melon; mixed nuts; corn tacos with fresh salsa; these and so many other fun items also create good health.

Choose well. Whether consciously practicing cancer prevention, undergoing cancer treatments, or altering your dietary habits following cancer, the good news is that the foods you eat may actually do you more good and make better financial sense than buying another insurance policy.

No one can absolutely guarantee that any particular diet will keep you from ever having cancer, but there's plenty of evidence that becoming really smart about food choices will put you in the winner's column.

One third of all cancer cases stem from tobacco smoking. Another third are attributed to poor diet. The remaining numbers arise from hereditary, environmental, and other causes.[3] Two out of three cancer cases, I believe, are preventable.

One third of all cancer cases stem from tobacco smoking. Another third are attributed to poor diet.

Most people experience far fewer and much milder side effects these days from radiation and chemotherapy treatments than ever before. Drugs and radiation techniques now used have become more specific. Also, new drugs can help combat nausea or fatigue that may occur.

Given this newer, far more level playing field, most cancer patients can easily adopt the nutritious dietary style we're discussing here. "Honey, I eat everything that's not nailed down," a vivacious Southern lady assured her luncheon companions. "I don't even notice that little old chemo pump they put on me." Watching her enjoy her crab stew, cornbread, and a lavish fruit plate made everyone else realize that cancer treatments aren't always the dreaded ordeals they once were.

Even when the big guns are brought out, it's still important to find foods you can tolerate and even enjoy.

Nutrition Despite Fatigue and Nausea

Perhaps there are times when a cancer patient really doesn't want to eat. That's the very time you should make the effort, our cancer survivors strongly advise. A piece of fruit, some crackers, tomato juice or vegetable cocktail, or applesauce, are all naturally good stomach settlers, and they also raise one's blood sugar to help lessen fatigue.

What you eat before treatments makes a lot of difference as well. One cancer survivor insists that a bowl of cereal

HINT

What you eat before treatments makes a lot of difference.

Choose foods carefully. Eat as wide a variety of fruits and vegetables as possible. Whenever possible, choose the freshest available. Keep your body well hydrated.

with low-fat milk made her chemotherapy much easier to accept.

Drinking plenty of pure water and green tea also helps. (Indeed, flavonoids in tea make it an excellent cancer fighter, according to nutritionists.) But be careful about the water you drink. I always recommend pure bottled water to everyone.

The goal is to eat well. Eat extra well, in fact. Choose foods carefully. Eat as wide a variety of fruits and vegetables as possible. Whenever possible, choose the freshest available. Keep your body well hydrated. (I only drink bottled water, both for its purity and because it's easy to measure how much I am drinking each hour and day.)

If nausea or fatigue should afflict you despite your best efforts, don't put up with such malaise. Ask your doctor to prescribe one of the new drugs that helps ward off such miseries, so you can return to the healthiest eating plan of your life.

Blue Ribbon Foods

All natural foods may be inherently valuable, but not all foods are created equal. For our purposes, we want to major in those with real star quality—those that get us on the fast track to good health.

Consider the following random list of nutritional heavy-hitters. Check your preferences. Are you getting enough of these foods and enough variety?

- Grains provide many vitamins and minerals, such as folates, calcium, and selenium, which studies show are associated with a lowered risk for colon cancer.[4]

- Low-fat protein foods: For quick energy and better mood uptake, three or four ounces of low-fat protein foods work wonders. Try lean, skinless chicken, fish, beans or legumes. Low-fat cottage cheese, tofu, or yogurt also helps.

- Carbohydrates such as organic cereal contain the amino acid tryptophan, which leads to production of a calming chemical called seratonin. As one woman reported, her morning cereal seemed to help prepare her against possible chemo-induced nausea.

- Maximize fiber intake by choosing a wide variety of whole grain foods: breads, cereals, brown rice, bulgar, crackers, pasta, and tortillas. Added fiber may fight breast cancer by decreasing estrogen levels in the body.

- Go for the gold. Deep orange sweet potatoes, carrots, rutabaga, winter squash, and cantaloupe are rich in beta-carotene.

- Pizza and pasta might not seem like cancer-fighters, but rich tomato sauces are especially nutritionally rich. Their lycopene-laden goodness is also found in guava, watermelon, and red grapefruit.

- Don't like broccoli? Eat the florets raw, dipped in plain yogurt, then sea salt. Cruciferous vegetables—

broccoli, cabbage, cauliflower, brussel sprouts—rate high on the cancer fighter's bonus list.

- Dark green, leafy vegetables like spinach, collards, kale, and Swiss chard are loaded with the phyto-chemicals that so efficiently attack free radicals.

- Citrus fruits: oranges and grapefruit. Can we possibly have breakfast without them? Not only refreshing and delicious, but nutritionally valuable.

- Berries: strawberries, blackberries, raspberries, and blueberries are all loaded with cancer-beating benefits.

- Dairy products: Use no-fat or one-percent fat milk. Some nutritionists suggest using organic milk from cows not treated with BST, a growth hormone, since there's a possible link to cancer. One or two servings of low-fat protein dairy products per day is suggested.

- Low-fat cottage cheese with flax seed oil is very nutritious.

- Soy products: Soybeans contain many compounds believed to ward off cancers. Tofu or soy milk once or twice a day gives you a broad spectrum of phy-tates, protease inhibitors, isoflavones, and other ben-eficial elements. Michael Milken has credited his use of soy products in helping fight off his late stage prostate cancer.

- Fatty fish: Omega 3 in salmon, white tuna, mackerel, sardines, and herring may help fight breast cancer.

These highly recommended, nutritional foods should appear on your plate two or three times a week.

- Tea: Think of it as a preferred-list veggie. Green tea especially provides extra jolts of flavonoids, but black tea also provides benefits.

- Wine: The marvelous heart-helpers and cancer-inhibitors found in red wine can also be obtained by eating red or black grapes or drinking grape juices. Alcoholic drinks do not mix well with cancer. In fact, more than one glass of wine per day for women and two for men may even cause cancer.

Monitor Your Servings

For once, you're urged to eat more: two or three servings of fruits and vegetables per meal, in fact. So what is a serving? Try these on for size:

- One cup of raw, leafy greens
- A medium piece of fruit
- One-half cup of cooked vegetables or fruit
- One-fourth cup of dried fruit
- Three-fourths cup (six ounces) of pure juice
- One-half cup of cooked beans or peas (black beans, pinto beans, kidney beans, lentils)

Concentrating on consuming small portions of a variety of these mega-nutritious foods not only boosts our basic health, but also provides other highly desirable benefits.

For example, a diet high in fruits, vegetables, and grains and low in meat, dairy products, and fat not only aids digestion and blood pressure, but also helps keep body weight under control.

Speaking of fat, we are advised to keep fat calories below twenty percent of our daily caloric intake and to avoid the hydrogenated fats found in cookies, muffins, pastries, and other snack foods. Medical opinions differ as to whether or not fats contribute to breast cancer. We do know, however, that they contribute to our waistlines!

Quality of Life

I have always lived life to the hilt, even during my breast cancer experience. I like good food and know how to cook it. But because I love life so much, no longer do I use the thick cream, sticks of butter, and calorie-laden gravies I once thought so desirable. Nor do I whip up those Dee Simmons chocolate chip cookie masterpieces (double chocolate, double pecans) I used to scarf down a dozen at a time.

No, we still enjoy good food at our house, but no longer do we push the envelope toward exorbitant, high calorie snacks, pastries, and other junk food I once adored. Look for high-nutrition gourmet recipes, and you can easily find them. Use your daily fat allowance to enhance those delicious vegetables: green beans almondine, for example, or buttered bread crumbs over fresh, tender asparagus. Dip whole wheat pita slices into a little virgin olive oil with scallions, rosemary, or other herbs mixed in.

The idea is, allow yourself to truly enjoy food. Become a vegetable and fruit junkie. Because of cancer, I broadened the variety of foods I normally eat and enjoy. I learned what was best for me to eat, and I learned to enjoy eating the very best.

Eat according to the USDA Food Pyramid, and your life will become healthier, wealthier, and wiser: healthier because you'll stave off illness; wealthier because extra energy and bounce makes you more productive and full of life; wiser because each day you are doing all you can to conquer cancer and stay healthy for life.

This may seem like a lot of discussion about food. Perhaps despite a lifetime of eating for health, you nevertheless encountered cancer. In that case I would encourage you to try the nine or ten serving fruit/vegetable regimen to increase your phytochemical intake and fight cancer-causing free radicals.

If you are eating right, don't stop—even if cancer treatments tempt you to slack off. And I'm not asking you to become a food fanatic either, someone afraid to ever nibble a piece of chocolate. But all the cancer survivors I talk to seem to emphasize the importance of becoming food prudent and knowledgeable about the powerful effects good food can produce on our body, mind, and spirit. This simply makes too much good sense to ignore.

Here is the good news:

- It's not all that hard to consume really health-boosting foods.

If you are eating right, don't stop— even if cancer treatments tempt you to slack off.

- A cancer experience can, and usually does, steer us toward the best foods for a better tomorrow.

- The mini-nutrition course in this chapter is easy to follow. For more detailed nutrition guidelines, see my Ultimate Living website, visit the internet, or go to your nearest bookstore.

- Pay attention to what you eat, and you'll begin to enjoy food more.

- Get those daily nutrition basics first, then relax a little when you're tempted to stray from the diet.

- You need not become a nutrition nut or health food groupie to eat better and improve your health with each meal you eat. However, I found my in-depth study of nutrition fascinating and absorbing. You may, as well. We all have a lot to learn about life, and what could be more basic to life than the food we eat?

A Personal Postscript

There's a precious and important postscript of my own cancer experience and subsequent delving into the study of food, nutrition, food supplements, and nutriceuticals. As I progressed in my studies, I never managed to interest Glenn, my husband, in all I was learning. "Just line 'em up and I'll take 'em," he'd say when I tried to sell him on the virtues of Green Miracle and other nutritional supplements.

Glenn was as good as his word. He did obey good diet guidelines, and he faithfully took the supplements I gave him. Unfortunately, this new outlook came along too late to stave off Glenn's eventual need for a quadruple-bypass heart surgery.

To everyone's astonishment, however, his good dietary behavior earned him a huge bonus in terms of amazingly rapid and uncomplicated healing, a speedy return to work, and the energy of a man twenty years younger than his age.

Like other cancer survivors I interviewed, I urge you to take a good look at your diet habits. If necessary, change your dietary ways—*today.* It is never too late, as Glenn and I can attest. And besides all the good food you get to enjoy, there are so many other health-boosters to consider: for example, nutriceuticals, exercise, relaxation, and spiritual and social outlets.

Stay tuned for even more be-good-to-yourself good news. Cancer survivors know a bundle of ways to get more life out of life—*every day* of your life!

Take a good look at your diet habits. If necessary, change your dietary ways— *today.*

MY THOUGHTS

Principle 3
Optimum Health

Can you put a price on good health? As every cancer patient learns, good health is priceless!

Promise yourself that during cancer treatment you will practice optimum health rules: the best nutrition, sleep, and exercise you can manage to provide. Ask a qualified nutritionist to advise you about food supplementation. Discipline yourself to observe excellent sleep habits. Decide to exercise each day in five or ten-minute increments.

Result: Enhanced health, fewer side effects, quicker healing, a better emotional state, and good habits which carry over into post-cancer good health for the rest of your life.

CHAPTER 7

BOOST YOUR IMMUNE SYSTEM

Like many other people today, I've become aware of the importance of doing everything I can to enhance my body's immune system. Admittedly, it took cancer to teach me to stay mindful of my natural defense system and truly respect this built-in life preserver.

Actually, it took very little study of the subject to convince me of two powerful truths:

1. Cancer, like so many other serious illnesses, results from lowered immune system defenses.

2. We are, as the Bible tells us, "fearfully and wonderfully made"—from brain to toes, each individual cell in the human body![1]

Is it possible to produce healthier cells and strengthen our immune system's functions? And if so, how do we go about it? Twenty years ago one of my friends asked her allergist, a noted specialist, those same questions. "There's nothing you can do," he told the middle-aged asthma patient. "The immune system wanes as the body ages; and yours is aging."

That statement, widely believed at the time, no longer is accepted as fact. It is true that one's immunity against bacteria, viruses, and chronic diseases may lessen over the years due to poor diet, tobacco use, lack of sufficient sleep, excess physical and emotional stress, and a host of environmental causes. Cancer, for example, is a long-term process; cell damage often takes place over decades before a tumor results.

Today a growing body of medical research provides overwhelming evidence that there's much we can do to avert the downhill slide of our essential immune system. During the past decade especially, many cancer survivors like myself have made it our business to learn what the immune system is, what it does, and how we can strengthen it.

We learn, for example, that when certain cells leave the thymus gland, their point of origin, they represent more than seventy percent of the lymphocytes coursing through our circulation system. Those T-cells, often called "killer cells," act as policemen sent to seek and destroy the bad guys: cancer and other destructive cells. Our job, then, is to make certain that we do everything possible to keep those T-cells at normal levels and working effectively. We now know much more about how we can help boost such immunity.

The job of cancer treatments is that of destroying tumor cells in the body by all possible means. The problem is, some normal cells get destroyed during the process. However, today's cancer treatments are making significant advances toward the goal of saving more good cells while isolating and destroying the bad ones. Modern medicine strives to keep the body's immune system working at as near-top speed as possible during cancer treatment.

You can imagine the complexity of that challenge. To meet such an enormous challenge, numerous centers devoted solely to treating and curing cancers today approach each patient's treatment in a totally individualistic way. Tumors are treated with the least invasive, least toxic, and least damaging strategies, using conventional medical therapies, beginning conservatively and stepping up dosages and procedures only if needed. Advanced cancers, of course, require heroic measures from the outset.

Blood analysis determines each patient's specific nutritional regimen. Such emotional interventions as medication, hypnotherapy, biofeedback, cognitive therapy, and prayer also become important treatment elements.

Does it work? Combining the best of conventional medicine with adjunctive dietary means and nutritional supplements, together with emotional therapies, often results in near-miraculously rapid cancer remissions and cures, according to oncologists and patients alike.

Mainstream medicine has begun to turn in the same direction, with growing numbers of leading hospitals, clinics, and research facilities presently conducting cutting-edge, cancer-related studies of the human immune system.

Alternative medicine, as most people call it, has become so well accepted that the U.S. government's National Institutes of Health several years ago created an Office of Alternative Medicine. More than thirty medical schools—Harvard, Georgetown, Duke, Columbia, and Stanford, among others—teach courses in alternative medicine, and the public spends some $31 billion per year on alternative treatments and health products—more than is spent on conventional medicine.[2]

Alternative, Integrated, Complementary

Though most people understand the term *alternative medicine,* it has fallen somewhat out of favor since "alternative" can mean "instead of" conventional medicine. "Instead of" might be okay for some maladies, but for such potential killers as cancer, it is highly advisable to seek the best, most advanced, and fail-safe treatments conventional medicine has to offer.

The alternative to alternative medicine, then, is what today we call integrative or complementary medicine—what I describe as the best of medicine combined with the best of nature. That combination, I am convinced, provides the most intelligent and effective route to supporting and mainstreaming our immune system, protecting it as much as possible so it can continue to protect one's body and life.

A major immunity safeguard is that of diet, as we discussed in the previous chapter. I don't mean an average adequate diet, but one crammed with nutrients and designed to vigorously fight off potentially threatening cells while it increases the numbers and power of our protective T-cells.

This requires diet supplements, as most agree—but only those that work at the cellular level. We will see how to choose the best of these for our purposes. And we will consider Michael Milken's persuasive arguments for soy products, nowadays so often a significant part of the breast, colon, or prostate cancer fight.

Increasing immune system functions requires other efforts as well. Sleep deficits play a role in lowered immune defenses as do such strong negative emotions as anger or depression. Obesity, overweight, and lack of exercise, all overly common maladies, also can weaken one's system.

More and more of us are turning to integrative, or complementary, treatments to help banish cancers and activate our immune systems. We are willing to try numerous alternative, non-medical therapies even as we actively seek the best new conventional medical methods. More physicians than ever before now advocate nutritional supplements, herbal remedies, relaxation, visualization, meditation, and prayer as valuable adjuncts to chemo or radiation therapy.

It might sound confusing, but those willing to explore complementary treatment options (after careful research of the many possibilities) and then decide how best to further enhance their healing regimen, have much to contribute to our understanding. No one advises embarking upon any complementary therapy, however, with which you might feel uncomfortable. And it must be stressed that substituting homeopathic, dietary, or other treatments for standard cancer surgery, radiation, or chemotherapy can be, and often is, fatal. Delaying conventional treatments to experiment with alternatives is alarmingly risky, since it allows tumors time to grow and metastasize.

What is the best approach? Cancer survivors list many ways they believe they boosted their immune systems and gained a cure. Like many, I continue to beat the drums for enhanced nutrition and a full array of dietary supplementation. Consider your body, with skin, hair, eyes, teeth, fingernails, joints and limbs you can see, plus intricately functioning internal organs and bones you cannot see, and you realize that the food we eat builds and determines the quality of each component of our physical make-up. No wonder I am so high on the importance of nutrition!

Health Without Risk

Medical motto: "First, do no harm." In the name of building a better immune system and fighting off cancer, some of us do some pretty extreme things—usually, of course, without our doctors' sanctions. I did a lot of experimentation, trying this or that potential remedy I'd hear about, and my doctor would warn me, "Just don't harm yourself, Dee, or spend a lot of money on pure quackery."

But that was before physicians and the lay public knew much about the effects of nutrition, food supplements, and a lot else that is common knowledge today. In those days I mostly went out on my own, contacting some of the world's leading research physicians I heard about, flying to other cities to interview them and obtain their recommendations. Much that I learned then in my own relentless searching is common knowledge easily obtainable today.

You can find a medical librarian to research your particular cancer, for example, and provide extracts from the most promising new medical research papers.

Yes, information can be obtained. You can make some wonderfully well-informed decisions. But there is one important caveat: Remember the distinction between becoming informed and proactive and self-medicating. Remember the physicians' motto, and adopt it for yourself: "First, I will do myself no harm."

REMEMBER

Remember the distinction between becoming informed and proactive and self-medicating. Remember the physicians' motto, and adopt it for yourself: "First, I will do myself no harm."

What To Ask Your Doctor

Always ask about dietary supplements and herbal therapies. Some of these may interact adversely with treatments he or she has ordered for you. Example: Dosing yourself with blood-thinning herbs before surgery.

Also ask about dietary restrictions or other guidelines. How much protein is advised? What kinds of fats should I avoid? What about caffeine and alcohol?

The idea is to rethink your approach to food, dietary supplements, and herbal therapies before undergoing cancer treatments, when occasionally even some ordinary substances might work against you. Example: Estrogen-high foods for breast cancer patients.

When we put on our full cancer-fighting armor, we are likely to start adding to our normal diet, health, and fitness routines. Most such decisions turn out fine. Many may be highly profitable. But for caution's sake, always consult your doctor or nurse assistant for advice. After all, your case is a team effort. Besides, they might know something important that you need to know.

Nutriceuticals

It is essential that we understand which dietary or nutritional supplements work at the cellular level. Those are the ones that can offer help early, before degenerative or chronic diseases get a head start. They are superb immune system enhancers. And in many cases, they actually reduce early tumors or heal lesions.

There is little doubt these days that nutriceuticals can play a powerful role in preventing and even reversing disease. Many scientific studies during the past decade alone have reported strong and convincing evidence to support the use of well-chosen nutritional supplements. Obviously, years of study have erased any doubts I may have had about their value.

However, I urge everyone to research the subject thoroughly before entering into a supplementation plan. Since each person's life, health-picture, metabolism, and disease differ from another's, we need to follow certain prudent guidelines.

1. Discuss your needs with a health care practitioner.

2. Beware of misinformation and false claims.

3. Consider carefully the quality of the supplements and the quality of the science that supports them. All supplements are not created equal!

4. Always tell your doctor about the herbals or vitamins you are taking. At times these can cause pharmaceutical side effects, just as prescription and over-the-counter drugs often do.

In summary, alternative, or complementary, medicine has gone mainstream in America. More money is spent on such treatments today than on conventional medicine. The billions we invest in dietary supplements alone show how serious we are about boosting our immune system, achieving better health, and living more nearly disease-free lives.

This encourages us to believe that with the best knowledge, wisdom, and supplementation, each of us can significantly enhance our health, thus helping ourselves and others in the ongoing fight to stamp out cancers.

REMEMBER

Before entering a supplemation plan:

1. **Discuss your needs with a health care practitioner.**

2. **Beware of misinformation and false claims.**

3. **Consider carefully the quality of the supplements and the quality of the science that supports them. All supplements are not created equal!**

4. **Always tell your doctor about the herbals or vitamins you are taking. At times these can cause pharmaceutical side effects, just as prescription and over-the-counter drugs often do.**

One Man's Decision

Michael Milken's personal fight against his advanced prostate cancer provides a stunning example of intelligent, proactive, and ultimately successful self-help. Cancer stalks silently, so when the famous young philanthropist and financier asked for a PSA test in 1993, it revealed a level of 25. Normal PSA levels are four and below. At the stage his symptomless disease had reached, patients usually live only another twelve to eighteen months.

Characteristically, the high-intensity young man plunged into a search for ways to cure his cancer. He decided to fight. Among the strategic decisions he made, lifestyle changes and diet in particular were the most immediate and dramatic.

As a college student, Milken says he never met a hot dog he didn't eat. Noted for his enthusiastic consumption of hot dogs and pizzas, the admitted "foodie" also liked daily breakfasts featuring bacon and egg sandwiches. A high-fat diet was built into his lifestyle.

Michael Milken nevertheless went on to beat his supposedly incurable cancer. He touts certain alternative treatments as central to his game plan. In addition to receiving conventional radiation and hormone therapies, he placed himself on a low-fat, high-nutrition diet. He believes one of his most important dietary changes was that of incorporating soy, which is associated with a lower incidence of cancers, especially those of the breast, colon, and prostate.

In a television interview with Barbara Walters, Milken, who lost not only his father but several other relatives to cancer, said, "I couldn't understand why every one of my family members lost their battle to cancer. Some had lasted a couple of years, some had lasted as many as eight years, but every single battle had been lost. My decision was that we had been too passive. The average person is too passive.

"Well, I just went to the library to check, but I was also trying to find out what I could do differently than thousands of other people I had spoken to who had cancer."

One major difference in Milken's approach was that of dietary change. He swore off high-fat foods and began to learn about nutrition. Convinced of soy's importance in fighting cancer, Milken eventually co-authored a bestselling cookbook, *The Taste for Living,* featuring recipes that incorporate soy and other healthy ingredients.[3] Proceeds from sales of this book and its sequel, *The Taste for Living World Cookbook*, support prostate cancer research.[4]

In the interview with Barbara Walters, Milken said he believes that he would have died of prostate cancer had he not changed his diet to include more soy products. He pointed out that Japanese men, used to a diet high in soy, have far lower rates of prostate cancer than American men. He concluded that America has five to ten times' higher death rates from such hormone-driven cancers as those of the breast or prostate gland than is common in other, soy-using countries of the world.

Facts about soy: Soy is the product of the soybean, one of nature's most highly nutritious vegetables. Tofu, also called bean curd, is processed from the beans. America's soybean production is enormous, in fact second only to that of corn.[5] It amounts to nearly 50 percent of the world's supply, yet Americans eat only about 4 percent of it. Ironically, most of our soybean production gets shipped to other countries where soy is regularly consumed, and where far lower rates of breast, colon, and prostate cancers are reported than those in the United States. Japanese men, for example, eat thirty times more soy than American men.

But soy, a scientifically proven cancer fighter and preventative, has caught on here in America. People are learning the value of soy protein and genestein, an antioxidant in soybeans, as cancer fighters and inhibitors. Perhaps largely due to Michael Milken's research and drum beating about soy, more Americans are learning its value and beginning to consume it. What's more, many doctors today believe that everyone with cancer should use such dietary intervention as part of their overall cancer therapy.

Why Natural Remedies?

Few people realize that many of the most potent pharmaceuticals in conventional medicine's vast arsenal simply relieve symptoms. They cannot eradicate the underlying ailment. For example, consider the common cold. We know there's no cure so far for this miserable malady, yet there are dozens, possibly even hundreds, of cold-relievers sitting on drugstore, supermarket, and variety store shelves. We spend millions of dollars per year on such drugs, which cannot, after all, cure our colds.

On the other hand, such herbal remedies as Echinacea are widely believed to boost the immune system, thus zapping the underlying reason for a cold. Not everyone can safely take Echinacea, many physicians argue, since some people are allergic to plants in the daisy family. However, not everyone can safely take over-the-counter pharmaceutical cold relievers, either. Read the warnings on the package before you assume their innocence and lack of side effects.

Physicians and patients in Germany, France, and elsewhere know Echinacea as a natural immune system enhancer and have numerous clinical studies which back up their beliefs.[6] Those beliefs have spread to the United States during the past decade or so, and today the native herb, which grows freely in most parts of our country, has become our number one bestselling herbal remedy in health food stores.

Europeans use Echinacea as an all-around immune system enhancer, whereas Americans usually take it to ward off their sniffles.

Plenty of other natural medications have well-proven scientific validity. None is a magic bullet, but American mainstream medicine, like that in Europe and elsewhere, has begun to accept and recommend plant-based diets, antioxidants, and vitamin supplementation, as vital elements of a multi-dimensional cancer program which complements the usual surgery, radiation, and chemotherapy.

Europeans use Echinacea as an all-around immune system enhancer, whereas Americans usually take it to ward off their sniffles.

■

One thing is for sure: anyone whose blood marrow has been suppressed by chemotherapy should seek ways to activate the body's desperately needed immune defenses. It would pay such patients to research nutriceuticals proven to succeed in rebuilding natural immunity—always, of course, with their doctor's knowledge and consent.

Such therapies usually prove less invasive, less harmful, and less expensive than pharmaceutical drugs. What's more, they work!

Other Immune System Enhancers

Step by step, we travel toward the realization that enhancing our immunity and basic physiological defenses requires us to see ourselves as whole persons—mind, body, and spirit—rather than just organs, tissues, muscles, and bones. The best cancer treatment centers, both conventional and alternative-oriented, recognize such truths and encourage patients to pursue healthier ways of thinking, relaxing, enjoying, and loving. It's eye-opening, really astonishing, for some individuals to learn that simply stopping to smell the roses actually helps boost their immune system and fights disease.

It's eye-opening for some individuals to learn that simply stopping to smell the roses actually helps boost their immune system and fights disease.

For others, such alternative therapies as visualizing cancer cells weakening, shrinking, and finally disappearing, learning basic relaxation techniques, or determining to eliminate harmful stress and toxic emotions from their lives become key cancer-fighting therapies. These methods of upgrading the immune system, once learned, should be used as a life and health enhancer long after cancer has been defeated.

One man said, "I had to learn how to be happy all over again. That was one of the most important parts of my treatment." Teaching ourselves to be happy, simple as it may sound, actually might just give us the healthiest immune system on the block!

Relaxation Techniques

Why learn to relax? Quite simply, here is your key to reducing stress, improving your immune system, and lowering blood pressure. Deep breathing, meditation, and exercise all help induce a relaxed state. Not only are relaxation exercises pleasant, but they are also helpful during various medical exams or procedures.

Five or ten minutes of deep breathing once or twice a day induces a deeply relaxed state which not only aids the immune system, but leaves you feeling super-oxygenated and refreshed.

Many people habitually cheat themselves of the oxygen they need by breathing short, shallow, stingy little breaths. Most people, in fact, could do a far better job of breathing than they do. Try the simple, beneficial exercise to the right and see how you feel. It could be a revelation!

Imaging, seeing something beautiful, enjoyable, and desirable, seems to come naturally once you achieve deep relaxation. Allow your mind to help you feel warm sunshine, hear enchanting melodies, or see a gorgeous garden or ocean view. As happy thoughts and images drift in and

"I had to learn how to be happy all over again. That was one of the most important parts of my treatment."

■

HINT

Deep breathing: Sit in a comfortable chair with your feet on the floor. Take deep breaths into your abdomen, and with your hand on your stomach, feel the relaxed muscles rise and fall as you pull oxygen into your lungs. That's all there is to it.

■

your mind and body become totally relaxed, your spirit feels the vitality and gladness of life. Despite cancer, pain, or any other illness, at such moments we can feel radiantly alive—and the immune system responds most positively.

There are other valuable approaches—exercise, for one, prayer, for another—which we will explore in later chapters, and which will add to the immune-strengthening process. For now, however, I simply want to emphasize the importance of making every effort to empower the immune system to kick-start or boost the body's built-in capacity to heal itself. Remember these facts:

- The human immune system can be strengthened and improved.

- It defends us against viruses, bacteria, common infections, chronic diseases, cancers, and other ills.

- We can activate the immune system by enhancing our daily nutritional intake and adding certain dietary supplements.

- Vitamins, minerals, herbs, and other natural remedies are important additions to cancer therapy, as many physicians and research scientists now know.

- Nutriceuticals are safe when chosen well and used appropriately.

- Never self-medicate with conventional pharmaceutical drugs or with vitamin or herbal supplementation. A health care professional should make sure your nutriceutical choices are pure and of standard dosage.

Your doctor should know of any natural drug you take in order to avoid adverse interactions with therapies that he or she is prescribing.

- The immune system responds to numerous kinds of therapies, including relaxation, acupuncture, visualization, exercise, positive thinking, prayer, imaging, and simple jolts of human joy.

Sick or well, make boosting your natural immune system a top priority. Investigate some of the ways to strengthen a so-so immunity or therapies that can help rebuild one that has broken down.

Dive into library research. Consult anyone knowledgeable about the immune system. Ask questions, seek new approaches, and above all, don't passively accept a cancer diagnosis.

When Michael Milken decided to become proactive, his life immediately changed. Combining conventional radiation therapy and hormone treatments with aggressive dietary supplementation and other alternative therapies resulted in his "incurable" cancer's retreat within *just six short months.*

Life is beautiful!

Facts About Our Immune System

- **The human immune system can be strengthened and improved.**
- **It defends us against viruses, bacteria, common infections, chronic diseases, cancers, and other ills.**
- **We can activate the immune system by enhancing our daily nutritional intake and adding certain dietary supplements.**
- **Vitamins, minerals, herbs, and other natural remedies are important additions to cancer therapy, as many physicians and research scientists now know.**
- **Nutriceuticals are safe when chosen well and used appropriately.**
- **Never self-medicate with conventional pharmaceutical drugs or with vitamin or herbal supplementation. A health care professional should make sure your nutriceutical choices are pure and of standard dosage. Your doctor should know of any natural drug you take in order to avoid adverse interactions with therapies that he or she is prescribing.**
- **The immune system responds to numerous kinds of therapies, including relaxation, acupuncture, visualization, exercise, positive thinking, prayer, imaging, and simple jolts of human joy.**

Principle 4
Boost Your Immune Defenses

Numerous medical research studies show that there's much we can do to enhance our body's primary defense mechanism, the immune system.

Presence of cancer or even the common cold shows a need to shore up our immune defenses. Some answers are better nutrition, exercise, and sleep. Beyond the basics, however, you'll discover a well-recognized world of complementary therapies known to boost immunity: massage, relaxation, neutriceuticals, visualization, deep-breathing techniques, and an array of other immune system enhancers.

Result: Seeking a variety of ways to boost immunity naturally makes sense to many cancer survivors, who advised us to stress two cautions: 1) Experiment only with therapies that you feel comfortable with trying, and 2) *never* self-medicate. Most survivors say they will actively seek to enhance their immune systems throughout their lives.

CHAPTER 8

EMOTIONS AND HEALING

We are emotional creatures; and few things in life can stir up stronger emotions than receiving a cancer diagnosis. Feelings of disbelief, sadness, and apprehension are likely to appear at once. Anger, really deep anger, afflicts many. "I felt my body had totally betrayed me," women often say.

And no wonder, when we have "done everything right," taken pains to stay fit, toned, and slender, worked out, eaten right, taken vitamins—and we realize that although we may look absolutely terrific, cancer lurks beneath the surface. No one who has not been dealt such a lethal hand can totally appreciate the feelings of the one who hears the C-word applied to himself.

HINT

"I felt my body had totally betrayed me."

Everyone I know who has dealt with cancer speaks to the emotional investment the disease requires. "First the news knocks you flat, and then you are urged to get your emotional act together. It's a tremendous psychological double-whammy," one man observed.

Everyone I know who has dealt with cancer, certainly each individual in this book, speaks to the emotional investment the disease requires. "First the news knocks you flat, and then you are urged to get your emotional act together. It's a tremendous psychological double-whammy," one man observed.

Behind such remarks lies the inescapable fact that now one must confront his own mortality. "I realized that everything I own is temporary," Tom Redmond said. Another man's first remarks upon hearing his diagnosis were equally poignant. "We've only been married two years," he told his wife with deep sadness. "But you will get well," she comforted him, and he did.

The stark realization that not just our possessions, but our life itself is temporary may shock some at first; but then, paradoxically, it brings many cancer survivors to a level of peace and purpose they never experienced before.

Physicians believe emotions both predispose us toward illness and also may play a highly significant role in helping us fight such diseases as cancer.

Emotions and Health

Physicians believe emotions both predispose us toward illness and also may play a highly significant role in helping us fight such diseases as cancer. Centuries ago Hippocrates said, "Man ought to know that from the brain, and from the brain only, arises our pleasures, laughter, and jests, as well as our sorrows, pains, griefs, and fears."

Today doctors believe that getting our emotional baggage out of the way, as one woman terms it, clears the physiological stage so that the immune system can do its best work. Though science cannot tell us exactly how emotions and the immune system interrelate, most doctors understand and agree that they do.

We all carry around some pretty mixed emotional bags: fear, depression, confidence, hostility, altruism, anger. You name it, and most of us have experienced it. Once an individual becomes a cancer patient, however, the winning strategy is that of siphoning off toxic emotions and strengthening the feelings which motivate us to persevere and win. The payoff, as Betty Rollin stated, is that "cancer made me wiser emotionally."[1]

Facing Feelings

The mind guides and directs our feelings. A woman's natural fear and dismay about losing a breast, a man's emotional state when he faces the possibility of impotence or incontinence due to prostate cancer, an elderly person's feelings about wearing a colostomy bag, all have to be dealt with, and the earlier the better. The cancer veterans I know offer some strong suggestions:

- Get the medical facts immediately. Understand what you are feeling about those facts.

- Ask plenty of questions. Explain to your doctor what bothers you most, and why. Ease your mind before you embark on surgery or other procedures.

REMEMBER

- **Get the medical facts immediately. Understand what you are feeling about those facts.**
- **Ask plenty of questions. Explain to your doctor what bothers you most, and why. Ease your mind before you embark on surgery or other procedures.**
- **Know about possible side effects before they can occur. Don't allow yourself to be ambushed by fever, nausea, weakness, or other physical effects that can plunge you into depression.**

- Know about possible side effects before they can occur. Don't allow yourself to be ambushed by fever, nausea, weakness, or other physical effects that can plunge you into depression.

- Chemo-induced hair loss can be traumatic for men as well as women. Don't delay deciding about cover-ups if your doctor tells you that medication will cause baldness. Do it now. A woman who heard the unwelcome news about her chemotherapy immediately bought a wardrobe of colorful turbans, scarves, and hats. "I started wearing them before I lost my hair, so by the time it happened, everyone was used to seeing me in them," she told me.

- Don't allow depression to linger. It is a luxury you simply cannot afford. Having the blues for a few days is quite understandable, but anything that lasts as long as two or three weeks may be clinical depression and must be treated.

- Don't even think about going it alone. Share your feelings openly with your spouse or one or two close and trusted friends. It is important to express your emotions and it is healthy to open yourself, perhaps for the first time, to receive feelings of caring, encouragement, and support.

Using your mind to explore, then deciding the parameters of your strong feelings will help guide you toward healing. As you approach treatments, here are some helpful principles to incorporate into your game plan:

- Appreciate your body's ability to heal itself.

- Think of your medical treatments as important allies—partners with your natural immune system.

- Explore the meaning of your illness and how it might change your life for the better. Example: Taking the opportunity to enjoy massage, stretching exercises, or relaxation techniques. "I explored everything that might help me," one man said. "Some of the techniques weren't for me, but others felt great."

Your mind will corral and capture your emotions as you work to understand and use them for your benefit.

Why Me?

We all ask that question, though almost certainly there is no concrete answer. Most of us never know why the wheel of fortune stopped spinning at *cancer.* But just as there is no point in continuing to ask why, there's absolutely no profit in blaming one's self or feeling shame or guilt over the disruption, heartache, and expense cancer creates.

Cancer is not your fault. You certainly did not sign on for it. It chose you. But if a cancer diagnosis causes you to silently and continually beat up on yourself in any way, grieve over what you have brought on your spouse, fear for your marriage, make you refuse to "spend your children's inheritance" to heal yourself—don't allow such feelings to go unchallenged.

HINT

Here are some helpful principles to incorporate into your game plan:
- **Appreciate your body's ability to heal itself.**
- **Think of your medical treatments as important allies—partners with your natural immune system.**
- **Explore the meaning of your illness and how it might change your life for the better. Example: Taking the opportunity to enjoy massage, stretching exercises, or relaxation techniques. "I explored everything that might help me," one man said. "Some of the techniques weren't for me, but others felt great."**

Many cancer survivors report the value of counseling to help them handle unruly feelings, large and small. Oncologists are accustomed to referring patients to psychotherapists to help overcome some of these overwhelming emotions.

Get the emotional relief you need, and be swift to reach out for it. Cancer, after all, is a big enough battle to fight. Your feelings of strength, power, and determination will help you fight the battle and win.

Depression

Though depression affects more than nineteen million Americans, two-thirds of them will never get help.[2] Those numbers are increasing, according to the World Health Organization, which estimates that by 2020, the incidence of depression will be second only to that of heart disease.

Cancer and clinical depression may be a natural combination, but one of them has to go if the other is to be successfully defeated. Treatments for clinical depression range from medications and psychotherapy to diet, exercise, stress control, and spiritual approaches. A lifelong, mostly unrecognized habit of "feeling low" might exist without our being aware of it. But serious depression can make an individual feel worthless, lethargic, hopeless, and unwilling to get out of bed in the morning. It depletes one's energy and appetite, and it affects one's relationships. Depression makes it hard to eat, sleep, or concentrate. You dread everything.

Obviously, depression-ridden individuals are not in peak fighting form—and cancer treatments require exactly that. If you recognized yourself or someone else you love from this brief description of clinical depression, contact your local mental health organization or ask your doctor to refer you to a therapist.

Such well-known personalities as Tipper Gore, Mike Wallace, Winona Ryder, and Deborah Norville have spoken publicly about their battles with clinical depression and the importance of seeking treatment.[3] A man I know told me he got furious every time his doctor advised counseling, but when he at last got to the point where his wife, physician, and others "ganged up on him," as he put it, he freely admits that therapy soon "changed his whole outlook for the better." He has beat four cancers over the past two decades, is presently in remission, and is working a heavy executive schedule. He also plays a mean game of tennis, dates his wife every Friday night (a new habit), and lives a happy life.

Those who resist treating their clinical depression, as this man did, often express great surprise at how quickly their emotional pain eases and their zest for life returns once therapy begins or medication is prescribed. If you or a loved one suffers from depression, run—don't walk—toward help. Get ready to take on the world again.

Emotional Stabilizers

Diet, sleep, and exercise are the three big factors that physically affect the emotions. Anyone whose glucose level

HINT

If you or a loved one suffers from depression, run—don't walk—toward help.

3

Keeping the blood sugar at normal levels with regular meals and high-nutrition snacks avoids the dangers of "sugar highs" or lows and does wonders for feelings of well-being.

■

drops precipitously can get moody, blue, irrational, fearful, or depressed. (That's why we reach for a doughnut when we should choose a piece of fruit instead.) Keeping the blood sugar at normal levels with regular meals and high-nutrition snacks avoids the dangers of "sugar highs" or lows and does wonders for feelings of well-being.

Simply paying back all sleep deficits is another way to boost endorphin levels, researchers say. A good eight-hour sleep habit helps make us immune to anxiety, short tempers, and depression. Sound sleep helps the body heal. Now, as never before, is the time to insist that you get it. Take a cup of herbal tea at bedtime and a good book or sweet music to fall asleep by, think happy thoughts as you drift off, and you should enjoy deep slumber.

Exercise, doctors say, rounds out the picture. Actually, researchers at Duke University Medical Center in North Carolina found that aerobic exercise did as much to relieve depression as medications and was easier to stick with. As little as fifty minutes of exercise a week cut depression levels in half, researchers discovered, and those who did more had even better results.[4]

While undergoing cancer treatments, you may not feel like running the Boston Marathon. But almost everyone can walk for ten minutes a day, five times a week. We can swim a few laps or plant a few flowers in the yard. It all adds up in the emotions department.

Exercise helps produce such "feel good" brain chemicals as endorphins and serotonin. Exercise can also be social, which adds to the benefits.

Those three basic physical components of healthy emotions—diet, exercise, and rest—make the best platform for peak emotional stability during a time that can seem like an emotional roller coaster ride.

Courage

The many examples of courageous approaches to cancer in this book have one factor in common: a rational response to the natural fears which crowd in when cancer strikes. As one cancer survivor declared, "I intended to live, not die." As it happened, her chances seemed medically iffy, yet she kept a good emotional head on her shoulders and eventually won. Today she handles a full schedule.

Procrastination always works against courage. It promotes fears and allows them to increase. Action and decision-making push us along during difficult emotional periods. Example: Choosing a wig early is a good antidote to a natural depression over having to wear one, former patients say. "There, I've done it" seems the most effective way to handle what for some is a big emotional hurdle.

Conquer procrastination and you steadily build more courage. Planning and acting on your own behalf knocks fear in the head. Knowledge about your medical condition

Three basic physical components of healthy emotions—diet, exercise, and rest—make the best platform for peak emotional stability.

HINT

Procrastination always works against courage. It promotes fears and allows them to increase.

and the disease itself and learning about all available remedies help you act with courage and intelligence.

Admit your fears. When a problem arises, speak to it. Acknowledge being afraid when that is true. Fear is normal, but talking about it and deciding how you wish to handle it puts you in control—and courage arises.

Courage can be learned. It can be practiced, as millions of cancer survivors have discovered. In fact, it is a revelation to get fully in touch with the overcoming power of our own human spirit. Learning to use our capacity for courage is a life-enhancing event.

Stress

At a garden center, two middle-aged friends greeted one another and began to talk. They had not been together for more than a year. "I had breast cancer," one explained. "Oh! I just got diagnosed with it last week!" came the reply.

The striking thing about that scene was where it took place: among long rows of growing, flourishing ferns, orchids, and beautiful bedding materials. One woman, treatments now completed, was there to decorate her garden and her life with fragrant stocks and petunias. The other, treatments still ahead of her, had come to find pleasure and take her mind off larger issues for a time.

Both women knew how to handle stress. Often a potential killer in its own right, stress should not coexist with cancer. Stress signals the fight-or-flight mechanism we are equipped with to mobilize the body. Continual stress keeps the body's systems in overdrive, shooting stress hormones into the system, which compete with and undermine our immune defenses. Worry, habitual overwork, anxiety, fear, and other negative feelings produce the stress that rushes the harmful chemicals through the system.

What counteracts harmful stress? A sense of control, according to researchers. Learn to handle your responses to events. Learn to adapt.

Some of the best ways to counteract stress will sound very familiar: breathing exercises, meditation, exercise, and nutrition. The value of deep sleep cannot be overestimated, research shows. With adequate sleep, things that usually bother us can be easily handled. That's why I believe so strongly in therapeutic sleep, both at night and during nap-times as needed, to make sure one is fully rested prior to any medical treatment, surgery, or other procedure.

Those workaholics who take a briefcase along when they enter the hospital have their priorities out of order, in my opinion. Their first order of business should be that of getting well. Lesser stuff can wait. Don't try to escape needed medical routines, but instead participate in them fully. You will be glad you did.

Again, never cheat yourself out of exercise. Even just ten minutes at a time—a walk around the block or a few minutes of stretching—helps abolish stress.

Caution: Always ask your doctor about the type and duration of any exercise you plan to adopt, especially during the weeks in which you may be receiving treatments. Of course, he or she should advise you about exercise following surgery. Your doctor will probably want you to exercise, but he or she also will want you to keep your efforts within sensible bounds.

Talk About Things

My feelings were all out on the surface. For some reason, I didn't expect breast surgery and reconstruction to be so painful. But confessing the, at first, nearly overwhelming pain actually helped. It made me realize that I am one of those people who can handle major pain pretty well. Talking, in that sense, helped me control my emotions, which, in turn, helped keep the pain itself under control.

Talking things out means you encourage yourself to think and act rationally—another source of control. The act of speaking about your plans and intentions, your worries and fears, helps your brain to assist you in organizing as you speak. And the more you sort out and organize life events, the more you are able to control strong emotions.

I don't necessarily advocate letting all your emotions hang out, even with your pastor, spouse, close coworkers, or certainly not with your child. Take your most unmanageable fear or angry feelings to a therapist. Short of that, however, talking about your cancer, your treatments, and your hopes and feelings about the experience with someone who cares about you not only puts your challenge into perspective, but also helps encourage the listener.

Journalizing

Some of us are intensely private people, and we really dislike the idea of sharing even superficial feelings with others. "I don't cry," one woman said. "If something is important enough to cry about, it's too important for mere tears." I'm not sure that a therapist would agree with that notion; most consider tears therapeutic.

But for someone whose tears remain permanently bottled up, journalizing might be a helpful emotional release. The brain, hand, and heart connect as we write, and troubles seem to flow through the ink and assemble themselves on the page—for your eyes only, to keep or destroy.

Intense feelings such as anger, hostility, or bitterness can be drained away by writing letters and then burning them. But the most productive way of expressing painful, difficult, or complex thoughts may be by keeping a diary. A written record of the ups and downs of a cancer experience not only is valuable while being written, but becomes an amazing record of personal perseverance, courage, fear, anger, resentment, and resourcefulness which can be reviewed in later years.

Date the entries. Write honestly. Record the revelations and exasperations. As you write, you will discover much about yourself that you did not know before. Cancer can

HINT

Intense feelings such as anger, hostility, or bitterness can be drained away by writing letters and then burning them.

TO-DO

Keep a Diary
Date the entries. Write honestly. Record the revelations and exasperations. As you write, you will discover much about yourself that you did not know before.

strip us down to the essentials, and it often reveals a lot about our own self-worth.

Keeping a journal helps drain away unwanted emotions and preserves the feelings you wish to remember. Like the feelings men say they experience during wartime, these are some of the most intense and true emotions you may ever experience.

HINT

A cancer diary is useful for recording dates, treatments, medical side effects and results, and names of physicians, therapists, and clinical personnel.

■

On a more down-to-earth note, let me add that a cancer diary is useful for recording dates, treatments, medical side effects and results, and names of physicians, therapists, and clinical personnel. Here is your record of a vital and life-saving time. It also contains the essence of your personality and character, which is well worth exploring and expressing. Value those pages and keep them for future reference.

People Who Need People

"Cancer helped me lose my inhibitions about saying simple, loving words. That made a major breakthrough in my life."

■

Be honest with yourself. Be honest with your doctors and the people closest to you in your ordinary life, your safety net. Such honest emotions as those that produce tears need no apology. Express your good feelings and even painful feelings to those closest to you, but control feelings of hostility, anger, and frustration. "I learned how to express the love I so often feel for people," a woman confided. "I always felt loving, but never before had I been able to put my feelings into words. Cancer helped me lose my inhibitions about saying simple, loving words. That made a major breakthrough in my life."

Cancer survivors, more than most other people, often seem more willing to share their emotions with others. Men who never before seemed verbal about feelings, now know how to express them. Instead of punching another fellow on the arm, they actually can say, "Man, I love you." That's really something.

If cancer does nothing else, it usually helps us learn how to unblock our emotions. This brings us closer to the rest of the human race. For that we can truly be thankful.

Healing Touch

When we feel uptight, stressed, and washed out in painful emotions, sometimes the mere touch of someone's hand can make suffering vanish. From centuries past, mankind has practiced healing by the laying on of hands. The Bible instructs us to do so, in fact, and from biblical times until today, the practice has persisted.[5] Touch accompanied by prayer often offers amazing relief, both physical and emotional, to a suffering person. There is something about the touch which conveys blessing and relief.

Most of us have held a sick and feverish child who is whimpering in the night, patting, and rocking, and cuddling the tiny body until the little one falls asleep, soothed by familiar hands. I believe we never outgrow the need for such hands and the therapy they can provide.

Somewhere I read that psychologists have established that we need fifteen hugs or touches each day to stay emotionally

HINT

If cancer does nothing else, it usually helps us learn how to unblock our emotions.

■

REMEMBER

Touch accompanied by prayer often offers amazing relief, both physical and emotional, to a suffering person.

■

HINT

Psychologists have established that we need fifteen hugs or touches each day to stay emotionally healthy.

REMEMBER

Find ways to give your beloved cancer patient more touching.

HINT

When attending the sick, I believe in laying hands upon the individual and saying a short, simple prayer. This can be said silently, said aloud, or softly murmured.

healthy. Science also teaches that babies deprived of holding, hugging, and touching fail to thrive. Elderly people have the same need. Often alone and perhaps feeble and no longer physically attractive, they seem almost to shrivel from lack of touching.

Enough said? From the cradle to the grave, human-to-human touch may be far more essential to well-being than most of us stop to consider. For a cancer patient or caregiver, that's something to think about. Learning to ask for a hug or a back rub might be a necessary step for some of us to take. A hand on a feverish brow can work wonders. Caressing a sick or suffering friend, child, or spouse helps us connect with them and ease a little of the anxiety we caregivers also may be feeling.

Find ways to give your beloved cancer patient more touching. This is one of the greatest emotional aids I know. Just the simple act of transferring your strength and caring to a tired or suffering person, connecting with them through loving touches—stroking, rubbing, or massaging—can work wonders. At age five, a kiss on the scraped knee makes it well. At age fifty, a kiss before or during chemotherapy also helps us heal. Is this really proven scientific fact? Probably not, but I have to believe hugs and kisses must boost the immune system!

When attending the sick, I believe in laying hands upon the individual and saying a short, simple prayer. This can be said silently, aloud, or softly murmured. During such moments, you can feel the person relax as the warmth of your hands and the good wishes from your heart seem to soothe and bring peace to the afflicted one. I believe such prayer heals. I have seen such holy touches work, and I have received them many times in my own life.

When It Is Someone You Love

Unless you married a saint or Superman, you'll become subject to a certain amount of emotional upheaval while your loved one experiences cancer. You want so much to help but can never tell where his or her feelings might be at any given moment. Cancer survivors offer some cogent suggestions:

HINT

"I got really tired of get well cards."

- Tom Redmond says, "I got really tired of get well cards." Other individuals echoed the sentiment, saying that they appreciated the thought, but something more personal and upbeat might help even more. A short visit, a phone call, an E-mail message, or a funny cartoon qualify as real uppers and help the patient feel normal.

- Try not to be Florence Nightingale. Treating the patient like an invalid is not always the best medicine. When Hal, who battled vocal cord cancer, resisted his wife's request for help with a small project, she said, "You're not all that sick. You just have a tiny little cancer, and the rest of you is healthy." Hal laughed, agreed to help, and they had fun all day. Her words, "all the rest of you is healthy," stuck with him throughout his treatments and helped him focus on the goal of healing.

- Silence is not always golden. When your loved one withdraws, gently attempt to coax him back into his normal ways of talking and acting. Don't challenge, but gently and patiently encourage him to talk about what is troubling him at that moment. Some of the most intimate times in any relationship occur when one partner is able to facilitate the other on a feeling level.

- Encourage laughter and light-hearted moments. Some physicians ardently believe in the healing power of laughter, and many hospitals find ways to encourage it. "Talking about the time our kid fell off the refrigerator made me laugh so hard, my pain disappeared," one man recalled. "My wife reminded me that when the doctor asked, 'Son, how does it feel?' he said, 'It feels like the time I fell off the tool shed.'" Laughing or flirting with a sick spouse seems to have healing value, releasing endorphins and making things feel normal again. Normal is good.

- Little surprises provide upbeat moments. Silly birthday hats, a sandwich made with the first tomato from your garden, or a love letter in the mail offer lasting benefits. Taking a box of candy to one's radiation therapist makes one feel more upbeat and in control.

- Practice your cherishing skills, but gently and not too obviously. Allowing the spouse to feel loved, special, interesting, and attractive provides an air cushion of good feelings which can help any of us to heal.

Feelings

Our feelings, like our words, create or destroy. Concentrate your attention on where you want to go, and your emotions will follow.

Guided by your mind and its intentions, even long-suppressed or negative feelings can be healthily expressed, then transmuted into powerful motivation toward healing and health. Yes, our feelings do help us heal, even from cancer. They are pure dynamite, and we should treat them with full respect.

MY THOUGHTS

MY THOUGHTS

CHAPTER 9

LOVE AND SELF-NURTURE

If love is one of the important seven principles for surviving cancer, self-love and the habit of good self-nurturing probably head the list. We can talk all we want to about the role good medicine, good thinking, and good nutrition may play in our health picture, or the benefits of massage, relaxation, and a positive mental attitude, but first we must value ourselves enough to put such ideas into practice.

Like most people I know, I thought that I took excellent care of myself. I stayed model-thin and always dressed the part. But maintaining an attractive or even a beautiful façade does not always demonstrate true self-esteem. Most of us in this fast-paced, striving American culture know how to look great and present ourselves

What we know too little about, though, is how to love and fully nurture ourselves.

well. What we know too little about, though, is how to love and fully nurture ourselves.

Love and healing play powerfully interactive roles throughout the course of every life. Lack of love undoubtedly inhibits healing, most would agree. But lack of self-love, a surprisingly commonplace malady, not only hinders healing, but often actually causes illnesses of every kind. For example:

- Allowing continual stress to compromise blood pressure, heart functions, hormone levels, and more

- Permitting years of being overweight to result in diabetes or high blood pressure

- Poor sleep habits, which cause everything from a bad temper to death due to highway accidents

- Taking such good care of healthy, athletic sons and daughters that there's no time for Mom to stay fit

- Ignoring doctors' advice or failing to take medicines as prescribed

- Neglecting to get regular mammograms, eye exams, or dental check-ups

- Failure to schedule colon exams and PSA tests

We are all guilty at times. "Too busy" is the usual alibi. But beneath it all, if we are honest, is the fact that often in our personal economy there simply is not enough love to go around. It certainly seems that way, if we always place our name at the bottom of the family needs list or leave it out of the family pot entirely.

Self-love

The value we place upon ourselves seldom rises high enough, psychologists say. Think of the people you know who honestly value not only their time, efforts, and success, but also their serenity, creativity, and peace of mind. Am I speaking your language here, or are you as out of touch with yourself as most of the rest of us are?

There's no deep mystery about the kind of self-love that can create a fully nurturing lifestyle. It requires no special expertise, no tremendous effort, and no excessive costs. But self-love and self-nurture are the twin principles that underlie all mind-body medicine. Properly nurturing one's self not only represents a commitment to excellent health and healing, but actually places something approaching a true value on one's life. It helps us practice good stewardship over the mind, body, and spirit with which we were endowed.

Beyond all that, self-love also forms the basis for the love and respect we feel for others. The Bible instructs us to love our neighbors as ourselves.[1] Only when I can love and value myself, in fact, can I offer others the kind of love I want them to receive from my life.

Cancer causes some of us to begin to understand the importance of learning to love ourselves. The idea at first may seem selfish; it may make us uncomfortable to think or speak about it. But at the bottom line, self-love represents our first step toward health, healing, and wholeness. We must do all in our power to foster it.

5

Self-love and self-nurture are the twin principles that underlie all mind-body medicine.

Learning To Nurture One's Self

The power of positive self-nurture can hardly be measured. It is a learned skill, and a vitally important one. Once we begin to put such precepts into practice, however, we not only improve and empower every aspect of our own life, but also set a standard for others around us to follow.

It may seem a little like learning a foreign language at first, but you can and should discover the benefits and joy of the following:

- Taking naps when you are tired or under par
- Connecting with the natural world by walking, gardening, boating, and other such activities
- Treating your mind to the finest music, books, and conversations
- Taking time for intimate friendship
- Expressing love to others
- Staying in touch with your emotions
- Dressing beautifully
- Choosing to eat only the finest, freshest foods
- Adding beauty to your life whenever possible
- Getting in touch with your senses

Take a look at the list (you may think of many other benefits as well), and you can easily see how self-love and a lifelong pattern of self-nurture contribute to keeping one's immune system at peak performance.

Believe me, the "selfish" habit of cultivating anything that works to one's best self-interest is the most *unselfish* way of life most of us could adopt. Good self-management, after all, is the key to becoming, as Benjamin Franklin said, "healthy, wealthy, and wise."

Too many people go through life feeling disappointed, cheated, downcast, or even abused by their circumstances. Self-love is the best prescription. It heals us and others around us.

5

Self-love is the best prescription. It heals us and others around us.

Self-Awareness

"Know thyself," a great sage ordered. "To thine own self be true," Shakespeare advised. But too often we don't love ourselves enough even to want to know our inner selves, and consequently, we fail to treat that inner person with due respect. Instead you should:

- Take time out of your routine to enjoy and appreciate life. (How many survivors of cancer do you know who say that at last they have learned to stop and smell the roses?)
- Believe you have a right to take time to pursue personal interests and things that give you joy.
- Don't feel guilty about doing anything that is not family or work related.
- Stop filling the empty spaces in life with sportscasts, TV sitcoms, shopping, or other diversions.

TO-DO

Assignment:

- List everything about your life that you consider unfair, non-productive, deficient, or painful.
- Write down ways to change each situation.
- Work on changing one thing at a time. The negative factors you listed could provide a road map to a better life, better health, and even, in some cases, a dramatic healing.
- Become self-aware. Treat yourself with the utmost tenderness, respect, and compassion.
- Realize that you are worth every bit of the effort, and much more. You have the right to pursue personal happiness and to live in full health.

- Don't feel guilty about spending money on such non-essentials as flowers or gifts.

- Refuse to live with chronic dissatisfaction or unhappiness.

- Stop giving every last ounce of devotion to jobs, care-giving for others, and similar responsibilities.

- Don't put up with perpetual boredom, fatigue, anger, resentment, or stress.

But Dee, you may ask, what does this have to do with surviving cancer? My answer is *everything*. Before considering health issues, we need to ask ourselves, "What kind of life do I want? What do I actually have?" Many can't answer these basic questions, but cancer survivors usually can. By facing one's life just as it is, with all its difficulties and deficiencies, it is always possible to change it. This is never selfish, but good for me and others around me.

Assignment: List everything about your life that you consider unfair, non-productive, deficient, or painful. Write down ways to change each situation. Work on changing one thing at a time. The negative factors you listed could provide a road map to a better life, better health, and even, in some cases, a dramatic healing.

Become self-aware. (I did not say self-absorbed.) Treat yourself with the utmost tenderness, respect, and compassion. Realize that you are worth every bit of the effort, and much more. You have the right to pursue personal happiness and to live in full health.

Plato's Prescription

"If the head and the body are to be well, you must begin by healing the soul," the philosopher Plato wrote. Doctors almost universally agree that there's a positive connection between emotional support and health. The trick is to learn how to support one's self emotionally and not always depend on such support from others. We sometimes need stronger inner tent poles rather than more outside props.

For example, support yourself emotionally before and during chemotherapy. A man I know always listened to tape-recorded show tunes and even hummed along. A teenager unashamedly brought along her childhood teddy bear. A woman wore rhinestones and sequins for a festive mood.

Self-nurture includes all sorts of things, including some, at times, that might seem slightly wacky. The idea is to focus on your needs and meet them with respect. If wearing rhinestones give you courage, by all means wear them.

It is at times like these—times of surgery and radiation, patience, fear, and waiting—that people so often rediscover a thrilling appetite for life. They do this by making every effort to heal their soul through assertive attention to their special personal needs, whether great or small.

Can a teddy bear heal a teenager? I say that if a beloved and well-used old bear can comfort someone and return her to a time of strength and joy, confidence and health, then she should go for it! You'll never find such advice in med-

HINT

Self-nurture includes all sorts of things, including some, at times, that might seem slightly wacky. The idea is to focus on your needs and meet them with respect.

ical books, I'm sure, but ask the youngster who tried it. She said it helped. Always ask yourself, "What would help me?"

Feeling Ugly and Undesirable

Face it. Having cancer attacks our vanity. Not only can the physical assaults of heavy treatments at times knock us flat, but changes in energy, weight, poor sleep, and other unwanted facts of life can convince us that we look terrible. Radiation therapy and drug treatments can make even the most incorrigible optimists believe their hair and skin and life as they once knew it might never return.

The antidote to feelings of ugliness and despair is to aggressively assert your self-nurturing skills. Now is the time for regular, even extravagant, pampering. Don't wait until this cruel war is over to fight back with facials, manicures, and massages. Do it now, and realize that hair loss, skin changes, and other ills will be kept at bay and damages minimized as you patiently minister to yourself in every way possible.

Give yourself time to recover.

Give yourself time to recover. Reassure yourself that all will be well as you perfect new health and beauty rituals and pamper your body and spirit in creative new ways. This is a healthy habit to form. And even when you feel not so hot, you'll enjoy yourself and feel your spirits rise.

Desire for Success

The couple looked as if they were about to be photographed for the cover of *Town and Country* magazine. He was dressed in white slacks and a polo shirt, white buck shoes, and aviator sunglasses. She wore white silk slacks, a navy blue silk pullover, a status scarf tied around her head, and a straw hat with a navy silk band tilted to shade her eyes. With her high-heeled sandals, gold earrings, and gold-rimmed sunglasses completing the picture, she would have ornamented anybody's yacht.

Safe to say, they were the best-dressed couple in a famous clinic's vast cafeteria. They seemed not to belong among the wheelchairs, sweat suits, and sensible shoes seen everywhere in the halls and waiting rooms, which probably caused all the stares.

Were they celebrities or movie stars? No, they simply made an effort to rise above circumstances. The woman who looked like someone vacationing on the Riviera actually was receiving treatment for widespread cancer. When her husband set her lunch tray before her, she smiled at him as though he were serving her pheasant under glass. As they ate and chatted together, they seemed worlds away from fellow patients in the same dining room.

The scene impacted others because the woman had dressed not for sickness, but for health. Where others looked neat and presentable, she looked knockout stylish. Watching from the corner of your eye, you could observe a couple who dressed well for one another. They took care to inject a little oomph into the outfit, and their upbeat attitudes reflected it. In a sea of sick people, they appeared perfectly well; yet her condition was as serious as most.

Do clothes make the man (or woman)? Yes, to a certain extent, I believe they do. Certainly nobody expects a cancer patient to dress as if a treatment equals a social event. However, if you observe those who dress up a bit, it's easy to see that self-nurturing seems to pay off in terms of energy and confidence.

7

Wear what makes you happy.

Wear what makes you happy. Wear clothes that make you feel attractive and well dressed. Avoid dull colors, too loose or too tight garments, or anything that feels harsh, scratchy, or uncomfortable. These suggestions can help you look and feel your best.

- Men look great in well-fitting jackets, shirts, and slacks. If you lose weight, be careful to find outfits that fit the new you. Save the too large garments for later. Sportswear is fine when it's well designed and snappy looking. Shorts, sandals, and T-shirts with messages are out, as are many other outfits that look as though you are about to rake leaves or clean the garage. When in doubt, ask your wife.

- Women should choose dresses or pants suits they'd select for business wear. Resist the temptation to wear anything floppy or sloppy. Good shoes, scarves, and jewelry do a lot for your look. At the end of the day, sturdy walking shoes with resilient soles help you deal with walking those long, stone-paved clinic or hospital halls.

- Choose head coverings with care. If baseball caps are not you, choose something with a bit more flair.

Colorful turbans, wigs, beautiful scarves, and hats made of soft velvet, velour, or lightweight straw can look quite becoming.

- Cancer centers often have cosmeticians who can style thinning hair or provide color and make-up advice. Skin tones can change somewhat or blotches can appear during treatments. Consult with an experienced cosmetician familiar with ways to cover rashes or soothe dry skin conditions. Learn ways to draw attention to your best features with new make-up techniques. Even if you consider yourself knowledgeable about such tricks, there's always something new to learn, and now is the time to learn it.

- Wigs come in almost every conceivable style and color these days, and in a variety of price ranges. Get fitted early, making sure you get exactly what you want before you need it. An ill-fitted wig can cause headaches. The right wig can provide self-confidence and a great sense of style, and many can fool even their nearest and dearest friends because the wigs look so much like the real thing.

Early on, decide how you will dress during your cancer experience. If you dress according to your mood, at times the results might look depressing. But decide how you want to look despite how you may feel, and your good looks can help boost even a sagging spirit.

Dressing well is an important component of self-nurture. It represents self-love in action and on display. Always

HINT

Early on, decide how you will dress during your cancer experience.

dress for your best image, that of good health and great success. All the rest will inevitably follow.

Your Private World

My friend Ann Platz, a prominent Atlanta interior designer, author, and speaker, also knows numerous practical ways to help surmount cancer. I asked Ann, who has family members who experienced cancer, to advise us on self-nurturing during an often lengthy period of treatments.

Ann strongly believes in the value and importance of good self-care. She says creating the right ambiance is essential to encouraging healing. "Chemotherapy often seems to heighten the senses and make the skin and nerves feel super-sensitive," she observed. "Everything the patient sees, hears, or touches should be soft."

"Everything the patient sees, hears, or touches should be soft."

Jangling noises, sharp tastes like lemon juice or tart apples, rough or scratchy towels, sheets, or clothing all distress those super-sensitive senses, Ann points out. "Think soft," she repeated. "Soft, soothing, and relaxing."

In particular, that translates into soft lighting. "Use three-way lamps for reading or resting, filtered light through blinds and curtains, whatever softens the room. I use pink bulbs in my lamps," she said.

Ann loves soft music and flowers in a convalescent's room, but she cautions against loud sounds or highly scented flowers. "An orchid is ideal," she said. "It is small, elegant, non-fragrant, and the blooms can last for weeks. A tiny vase with a few garden flowers or a single perfect camellia or rose also make good choices." Ann Platz is noted for her color expertise and has strong opinions about how color affects well-being. Light, pure wall colors, and pretty colored bed linens and bath essentials are the rule, she says. "I love pink and always choose pink lingerie, bedding, and towels," she told me. "It's a color that's both soothing and flattering to most people. Men usually don't object to pale pink," she added.

Ann told of visiting a friend who was hospitalized. When she asked the woman if she could bring her something she wanted or needed, the patient implored her to bring some soft sheets. Sheets with an extra high thread count matter a lot to someone whose sensitive skin is irritated by rough fabrics, Ann points out. She says bath towels should be rinsed in double amounts of fabric softener, and old, soft, well cared-for sheets and pillowcases should adorn the bed.

Bedclothes should be not only soft, but also as lightweight as possible. "The weight of bedclothes and softness of sheets is so important to anyone whose skin is sensitive from radiation therapy, chemo, or long stays in bed," she warned.

Following is Ann Platz's prescription for making the perfect bed to comfort a cancer patient.

- Use several lightweight layers of covers. Featherweight blankets and ultra-soft sheets and pillowcases are a must. Satin or down pillows feel smooth and luxurious.

- Place a feather bed over the mattress. This feels as though you are resting on clouds. Use down-filled pillows of various sizes and firmer pillows to support the back. Place baby pillows beneath the neck, elbows, or any place that feels sensitive from lying in bed.

- Use a fitted sheet above the feather bed, then double sheet the top layer. That is, place a lightweight blanket between the two top sheets for utmost softness, warmth, and comfort.

- The bedspread, if any, should be very lightweight. One should never sleep beneath the spread, but it should be folded at the foot of the bed when the bed is occupied.

- Silk or mohair throws add still more warmth and softness, and they are for the patient to arrange around himself for maximum comfort.

Other Practical Comforts

A bedside table or nearby chair can hold such must-haves as photos, a lamp, tissues, and reading glasses. Place baskets nearby for reading and writing materials, the remote control, and the like. A basket filled with rolled-up fingertip towels can be quite useful and welcome.

Nightlights, softly scented candles, and such sentimental objects as pictures or photo albums bring happiness into the room, as does a selection of happy audio and video tapes and perhaps a nearby bed for one's pet.

With a little thought and effort, it's possible to turn a bed, even a hospital bed, sun porch, or any other nook, into a space of special pampering, beauty, and comfort—a perfect place to regain one's health.

"I believe in making every room in your house just that wonderful," Ann declares. "I have soft lighting, soft seating, and soft colors, music, and flowers throughout my home. I placed featherbeds over each mattress. I believe in comfort and restoration for everyone, not just those who are sick."

"Illness strikes without warning," she continued. "That's usually not the best time to properly furnish a sick room. Make your entire house encourage well-being, and do it *before* anyone gets sick."

Take a leaf from Ann Platz's wise book, and make your entire home a place of self-nurture for everyone in the family. Such efforts will nourish you in every way, adding joy, health, and well-being to your life.

The Power of Love

Love and pleasure work together for healing and good. Love yourself enough to nurture yourself well, and from your wellspring of daily contentment, you will find yourself better able to pour healing waters over everyone you encounter.

If cancer teaches us nothing else, it certainly shows us the importance of all life—including our own, which we so often overlook and neglect. In our pathway back to health, two roads must be taken:

Love and pleasure work together for healing and good.

HINT

1. Learn to love and nurture yourself well. Make a lifelong commitment to that principle.
2. Look forward to a lifetime of loving, sharing, and nurturing others as well.

1. Learn to love and nurture yourself well. Make a life-long commitment to that principle.

2. Look forward to a lifetime of loving, sharing, and nurturing others as well.

The force of love not only plays a powerful role in our healing from disease, but also transforms all of life. Love yourself tenderly. Forgive your faults and blunders.

Find ways to cherish and celebrate the good you see in yourself and all that you love in others. Always remember, the love, empathy, and acceptance we offer ourselves, thus providing good treatment, results in our outpouring of good to others around us. Learn to love yourself well, for the sake of everyone else in your world.

MY THOUGHTS

Principle 5
Love More

Emotions may predispose us towards disease, doctors believe, or help us battle serious illness. Healthy emotions steer us towards healing and health, most medical experts agree.

Love exerts a powerful force in the healing process. Self-love leads us to respect the person we are enough to give ourselves the best possible care, and treatment, and to believe in our power to prevail. Giving our love to others and receiving their ministries, care and affection in return not only boosts the immune system, but also gives us the will to fight.

RESULT: The well-loved individual possesses one of the most potent healing effects known to the medical profession. The more love, the better climate for healing.

CHAPTER 10

MORE LOVE,
MORE LIFE

When Sarah mentioned to Phil that she could hardly wait to leave the hospital and "veg out" on their leafy backyard terrace, her husband had a great idea. He headed straight to their local garden store to put his plan into action.

The next day Sarah, weak and tottery but thrilled to be home, walked with Phil to their terrace. Startled, she looked around then squealed with delight. "Phil! When did you do all this?"

Pillows, a throw, and a cluster of balloons adorned her chaise lounge. But it was the six freshly planted rose bushes perfuming the air, the new hummingbird feeder hanging from a nearby tree branch, and a newly installed bird bath already teeming with customers that made her catch her breath.

"Honey, you shouldn't!" she exclaimed, but Phil shushed her. "I don't want you out here by yourself," he kidded, as a pair of squirrels streaked across the lawn, "and I've got to go back to work."

That was several years ago. The rose garden has expanded each year since. It requires a lot of time and work. But each rose reminds Sarah that Phil loves her, understands her, and sticks by her through thick and thin. Her fierce battles with cancer are long since over, but an adoring husband and the perfume of roses remain.

Busy these days with a fully packed schedule, Sarah nevertheless manages to escape for an hour or so each day to her "quiet place" with a book and her thoughts. Sometimes she and Phil have a glass of tea and chat; other times he works with the roses. Life is good, as this small, beautiful piece of the world always reminds them.

The love principle is almost always the first thing survivors speak of when telling others about their experiences with cancer. I have heard any number of love stories from them, and they always make me smile. The hospitalized mother whose three grammar school sons wrote a book for her concerning their family life, printing the text in crayon—the stories so unintentionally funny, she said, that they made her laugh and cry. And a man receiving cancer treatments at a facility in another state who wanted his wife to stay home with their infant daughter proudly said, "I

The love principle is almost always is the first thing survivors speak of when telling others about their experiences with cancer.

received a love letter from her and the baby every single day I was gone. I still have every one of them. I'll give them to our little girl when she grows up."

The fight to live arouses in most of us an equally fierce need to give and receive love. This can challenge all involved. The patient, as we said earlier, may well be confronted with the unfamiliar challenge of needing to learn how to love and nurture him or herself. This might not be easy for some. The patient's family, meanwhile, may need to learn new lessons in creative cooperation. The healthy spouse seeks ways to express love to the afflicted one, and to empathize, help, and "be there for him."

Love and Healing

Without any doubt, love helps us heal. Doctors observe the potent effects of the connection between love and medicine. Physicians remark, in fact, that they'd much rather shoo an overflow number of visitors from a hospital room than enter a quiet room where a patient lies motionless, with his face turned to the wall.

Without question, I believe, love ranks as necessary to healing as any amount of clinical expertise, state-of-the-art treatments, or the newest drugs or surgical techniques. When we are sick and scared, we need love, and lots of it. Even the most buttoned-up, non-emotional, matter-of-fact, macho guy you know will come to the end of that attitude the moment the C-word is applied to him. Human love,

The fight to live arouses in most of us an equally fierce need to give and receive love.

When we are sick and scared, we need love, and lots of it.

touch, care, and the willingness to put feelings into words matter desperately to the patient at such a time.

For the friend, sweetheart, or family member, it becomes terribly important to find ways to show love to someone we treasure. You furtively size them up, wondering how much expression is too much, how to keep from saying something inappropriate or embarrassing, or even how to keep from bursting into tears.

The need to express love to another, the conviction that you must do so, arises again and again. It can actually make us uneasy and at times create anxiety. But somehow we learn ways to reach out beyond our usual emotional boundaries, stretch a hand toward the one we care so much about, and figuratively pull him or her away from cancer's illness, fear, and depression and into the safety and promise of normalcy and health.

The good news is, our love, far more than we can imagine or measure, helps us do just that. Clumsy as we may believe ourselves to be, some days the simple love we offer works miracles.

Men and Women

At no time do the differences between males and females show up more sharply than when we become sick. Trust me, we handle everything from cancer to the common cold in totally different ways.

For example, it surprises me that so many men admitted that they really disliked receiving get-well cards. I simply could not figure that out, until one friend explained. "They remind me that I'm sick. I have cancer."

As far as I know, that's mostly a guy thing. Men often despise the idea of sickness. Lying in bed, feeling weak, losing weight or muscle tone, being temporarily unable to work out at the gym—these sorts of things are contrary to the macho male. Add a greeting card with a happy face to that syndrome, and the love message you intended to convey might not be received as you intended.

Send the same card and the same mushy sentiments to a female friend, however, and you're likely to receive a far different reaction. Survey your mother's or girlfriend's bedroom or hospital room and you'll see greeting cards propped up on every available surface and even pinned to the curtains. She is delighted with her cards and reads them over and over.

Whether male or female, the same love motivates us to reach out to those with tough battles ahead of them; yet all cancer patients are not alike. A grandfather needs as much love as a high school football quarterback needs, but different expressions may be appropriate. Women, on the other hand, usually are far more in touch with their feelings, doctors observe. Used to nurturing others, they easily slip into the role of caregiver or recipient.

My job as a friend, spouse, or neighbor is to intuit, as far as possible, the best ways I can relate to my cancer-stricken friend's need *at that moment* and offer whatever physical, mental, or spiritual "medicine" I can. This may be as simple as a hug or kiss, anticipating a need and running an errand, listening to her feelings and responding with a perfect word of encouragement, or offering to pray for her quietly, out loud, then and there.

For any of us who so deeply desire to help another person regain his or her health, finding ways to put love into action becomes a life-enhancing adventure for the giver. For the patient, learning to receive love often teaches life lessons he or she will never forget. Each partner in any love exchange rediscovers some powerful truths: We all are inter-connected in this life. Commitment to serve others always enriches us. And, as the Bible says, "Love never fails."[1]

These are humbling, inspiring, unforgettable lessons cancer teaches us. The word *privilege* often crosses our lips. The opportunity to love, serve, and commit becomes holy and treasured.

What Love Does

"In sickness and in health" takes on a whole new mean-ing once cancer strikes. How will others stand by us, we wonder, accept us as we are, and help us through something we absolutely never planned to take on?

We may never put such feeling into words, but they are there. *Is our sex life over?* is the thought that crowds in late at night, when the hospital is quiet and we're too restless and disturbed to sleep. Or, *I need to go back to work, but I dread having to wear this wig.* We feel so vulnerable, and our feelings surface at such unexpected times.

We may wonder if our marriage has changed—somehow become less of a partnership and more of a care-giving situation. And how much have we ourselves changed—permanently? Will we still be perceived as a ball of fire, or as a sick person? Will we still be accepted, or is who we really are now vanished forever?

Here's where love, loyalty, and commitment can come crashing through. Story after story of people's magnificent abilities to empathize, meet another's need, and sometimes even sacrifice for the sake of love prove that, inept as we may believe ourselves to be, we were created and have been programmed to love one another. Don't think you won't be able to love your dear one well. I know you can, because that ability was installed in your wiring when you were created. You arrived with the blueprint in place. Now you can use that potential to its fullest, and, in so doing, vastly expand your capacity for reciprocal love. It can seem almost miraculous.

Once they understand such capacities for love, survivors tell me, it alters their lives forever. I know my own compassion for anyone struggling with the pain, fear, and sickness cancer can bring. I want to do everything in my power to help them surmount their suffering and survive. That empathy never wanes, as one cancer survivor after another testifies.

5

Once they understand such capacities for love, survivors tell me, it alters their lives forever.

Cancer opens the floodgates of your love. You know its power because you experienced it. You lived, and you want your brother or sister to live. So when you go to them, counsel them, hold their hand, or simply sit at their bedside for a night, you know that even under sedation, they can feel the love extended toward them, the love that surrounds them and fills the room.

There's a well-known story about former First Lady Betty Ford, who had breast cancer surgery soon after President Ford took office. She was one of the first influential breast cancer patients to go public with her story in hope that other women would be encouraged to get a mammogram. Mrs. Ford asked her husband to come to the hospital during her bath time. She wanted him to see the now flattened side of her chest with its fresh scar. "Would you love me any less if I lost an arm or a leg?" the president asked.

That day it was not the President of the United States who sat at the First Lady's bedside, but two hurting people who extended encouragement to each other. The devoted couple's marriage has lasted some sixty years.

People Who Care

I'm always amazed at some of the creative ideas loving people can dream up. Phil's rose garden, for example, not only celebrated a special moment, but has lasted to this day. I asked several cancer survivors to share their favorite love stories for this book. (In most cases, names have been changed.)

"I love opera and was undergoing chemotherapy when a performance I really wanted to see came along," Alex told me. "I was pale and skinny and had just lost all my hair. Going out in public was totally out of the question. For one thing, I was too weak."

But Alex's wife, Nancy, and another couple decided live opera might be just what the doctor ordered for Alex. They got special permission for him to be seated backstage, reasoning that he could leave after the first act. After some negotiations, the director gave his permission, outlining with tape the space where Alex could view the opera from the wings.

The director had bent the rules for Alex, and Nancy and his friends hoped there would be no repercussions. At first Alex was dubious about the scheme, but at last agreed to go along with it. After all, the three had gone to so much trouble for his sake, and one act shouldn't exhaust him, he decided.

The evening proved gloriously successful. Backstage activity fascinated the opera fanatic, and his vantage point from the wings allowed him not only to enjoy the full power of the performance up close, but also to view the audience's reaction. Alex was stimulated and enthralled.

Between acts, among scenery shifts and costume changes, famous singers made a point of stopping and talking with Alex. The patient ended up staying for the entire performance, for an evening he will never forget. Happy and exhilarated, he thanked his companions again and again. He believes his healing from a difficult cancer began that evening. Today he is well and happy, and he enjoys grand opera more than ever before.

—

A yearly reunion of several college sorority sisters, now in their sixties, seemed doomed when Mary Ellen had to have cancer surgery shortly before they were to meet at their favorite beach retreat.

Should they call off the reunion and wait until next year? It wouldn't be the same without Mary Ellen, they all agreed. Plans and logistics hung in mid-air for several days as the friends consulted with each other. Finally it was decided that one of the "girls" would drive to Charleston and bring Mary Ellen to the beach. (No husbands allowed.) They would feed her, love her, walk with her on the beach, and encourage her in every way old friends know how to do.

Selfishly, each knew their entire week's rest and relaxation would be given to Mary Ellen's needs. Unselfishly, they decided they wouldn't have it any other way. So they fetched the patient, who was well loaded with doctor's instructions and emergency phone numbers, and tried to place everybody in their customary fun mode.

A week of bridge games, banter, seafood suppers, jokes, and ceaseless talking went forward as usual. The girls took Mary Ellen to the beach early each morning before it got hot and crowds began to arrive. They made her take naps.

Nobody smoked cigarettes that week, or got too noisy, or squabbled about anything at all.

"It was beautiful and unforgettable," Mary Ellen says five years after her special holiday. "They refused to leave me out. They came and got me, gave my poor, old husband a week's rest, and then drove me back home. By the time I was ready to begin chemo treatments, I was up for them. My friends gave me such confidence."

The girls still have their beach reunions. "I'm their big success story," Mary Ellen brags. "I lived, and the girls are so proud that we all stuck together that year. We would do anything in the world for one another."

—

Jason, a strapping seventeen-year-old sports jock who excelled at both football and basketball in high school, became sidelined with leukemia. Chemotherapy left him weak, uncharacteristically dispirited, and totally bald.

"One day his football teammates all trooped into our house to see him," his mother said, "and every one of these kids had shaved his head. We had the biggest round of high fives and loud jokes going on that you've ever heard under one roof! Jason was amazed, just totally freaked out. Soon he was sitting on the bench at every game, cheering and kidding the other guys. His oncologist said he couldn't believe how fast Jason got well after that. He was always a healthy kid, but I believe his teammates' support did even more good than all the medicine!"

Such stories are typical of the many ways love extends a helping hand. Sometimes you see love in action when you leave home—little snapshots on the street: a frail, elderly woman in a wheelchair whose granddaughter is wheeling her through the mall; a skinny young man in a baseball cap enjoying a fast boat ride and cheering his buddy riding on water skis behind him.

Once you've had cancer, you're alert to those little love scenarios. You smile, and you say a little prayer for the granny someone is helping to shop, or for the fellow in the baseball cap.

Love Gifts

We all love to receive gifts, especially when we're sick, but when you choose a gift for someone who is seriously ill, please stop and think. Large, fragrant bouquets may be beautiful, but they are out. There's not enough bedside table space, for one thing, and the scent might induce nausea, for another. Candy is usually not desired. And books can be hard to hold when you are weak, and they take too much effort to read when you are tired.

So what *do* cancer patients enjoy? Stacey appreciated her girlfriends' taking turns sitting beside her hospital bed, quietly reading or doing needlepoint. She could doze or chat as she felt like it. There was always someone to rearrange her pillows, bring her a cool drink, or help her to the bathroom. She felt loved and secure.

—

Norah's office mates took turns bringing dinners to her house throughout her long illness, freeing her husband to take care of their children.

—

Marian asked her neighbor to plant the tulip bulbs she had stored in her refrigerator. "That meant so much to me," she said. "She planted, mulched, fertilized—everything. They were just beginning to bloom when I finished my final treatment."

—

Ed's friend, also his attorney, reminded him of his tax returns, helped him collect needed paperwork, then carried it all to Ed's accountant. "That was real love," Ed joked, "keeping me out of jail."

The best thing you can give a sick relative or friend is yourself.

The best thing you can give a sick relative or friend is yourself. Offer to drive the patient around the neighborhood to see the Christmas lights. Carry their garbage to the curb. Show up with a big bowl of salad or a hot casserole. Take their clothes to the dry cleaners. You can think of a hundred ways to give love that will be more useful and appreciated than a fruit basket.

Frieda Courson gives a moving account of the day she had a lumpectomy procedure and was given a cancer diagnosis. "For years I had prayed I never would have cancer," she said. "Other family members, especially my sister Bobbie's husband, had endured terrible cancer experiences.

I took good care of myself and hoped and prayed I never would follow in their footsteps."

The day of her surgery, several close friends drove into town to be with her and her husband, Tom. "One friend, who stays overwhelmed by the needs of her ninety-year-old parents, drove from Chattanooga to Atlanta to be with me. My sister Bobbie flew up from Florida. Another friend with severe heart trouble found someone to drive her from Alabama. There were others who lived close by.

"Soon after the surgery, my news arrived. *It was cancer.* To my own great surprise, I felt no fear, despair, or any great disappointment. There were no tears. I felt total calm and perfect peace. The love and prayers which surrounded me that day bore me up like an air mattress. I cannot adequately describe the feeling. I can only tell you that I have experienced the power of perfect love."

Another story that touches my heart concerns one husband's reaction to his beloved wife's illness. "A highlight of her experience was our joint decision that we would hold musicals for just the two of us each evening, using our own rather extensive record collection. We would play all the Brahms, all the Mozart, and all the Puccini we possessed, in the order in which they were composed.

"It was a tremendous intellectual and emotional trip. Nothing brings you much closer than sharing great music. Music literally heals your soul."

That man gave of himself. He gave time, gentleness, love, involvement, understanding, and encouragement. The gift of such devotion helped both to heal.

Plan To Love

Decide to love the sick. This represents an active decision. Here are some things cancer survivors hope you will remember:

- Your love is needed and essential.

- You are a part of the patient's healing process.

- Follow your heart.

- Be willing to schedule time to do the small tasks, which mean so much.

- Do small tasks with great love.

- Gentleness and quiet companionship are like a soothing balm.

- Love boldly. Do not fear rejection.

- Write one or two-sentence love notes to hide in books, drawers, or bathrobe pockets for your loved one to discover. My mother wrote hundreds, perhaps thousands, of these to me.

- Read aloud. Choose beautiful, short, inspiring passages.

- Smile often. Gently touch your loved one's skin, hold his hand, or smoothe her hair. Stay connected.

MY THOUGHTS

CHAPTER 11

FAITH AND HEALING

Story after story, including my own, illustrates how important the Faith Principle becomes once cancer so rudely invades our life. Just as soldiers say there are no atheists in foxholes, I believe you'll find very few in oncology units. When cancer attacks, people like Frieda, Hal, Destinae, Tom, and thousands of others arm themselves as the apostle Paul instructed, with the shield of faith, the helmet of salvation, and the sword of the Spirit.[1] We desire to fight by all means possible and to win.

These days modern medicine has begun to recognize and study the correlation between physical and spiritual health. Such individuals as Joe Gagliardi, who recently headed the Cancer Treatment Centers of America in Tulsa, believe that "faith is a strong element that needs to be harnessed in the healing process." Several cancer survivors in this chapter describe ways they utilized their religious faith during every aspect of their recovery process.

The human physical-spiritual link is an age-old concept.

The human physical-spiritual link is an age-old concept. For eons, mankind has instinctively believed that physical and spiritual health are intertwined, but during the past two centuries, Western medicine veered away from such beliefs and placed its faith in pure science. Science certainly rewarded us with important medical findings during the past several generations, with many advances discovered during our lifetime. In the past decade alone, cancer diagnoses and treatments in particular have become increasingly more sophisticated and successful.

But in the two centuries during which *medical science* marched forward, non-laboratory-tested *religious belief* became increasingly less important in the practice of "good medicine." Indeed, in many scientists' minds, faith and medicine seemed mutually exclusive.

These attitudes are changing. Today's double-blind research studies and ordinary blood tests actually can measure the beneficial effects of prayer and religious belief on an individual's immune system. Along with medicine's fabulous advances in technology, drugs, state-of-the-art surgical procedures, new vaccines, and ongoing research, factors of faith and prayer are being added to the healing equation.

Polls repeatedly show that most Americans profess to have at least some degree of religious faith.

Polls repeatedly show that most Americans profess to have at least some degree of religious faith. A high percentage regularly attends church or synagogue. The overwhelming majority of us say we believe in God. A cancer diagnosis, therefore, means that most of us instinctively reach into our faith resources. Issues concerning mortality lead us to review core values and beliefs. We examine our inner selves. And when we feel sick, scared, vulnerable, or alone, most cancer patients will look even to the simple faith of their childhood as they grope for answers and help.

Faith Makes Medical News

In recent decades, scientific attitudes toward faith and healing have become increasingly more open to inquiry. Today many of our nation's 125 medical schools include in their curriculum such courses as comparative religions and their teachings about healing.

Meanwhile, internet chat rooms and religion-based web sites offer information and personal accounts of faith and healing. Hospital and community-based cancer patient support groups often include prayer, healing Scriptures, and meditation in their programs. Anyone can add a name to prayer chains in which people pray daily for the individual by name until he or she considers medical treatments and healing complete. Some of these chains of believers we will never meet for they reach into countries far beyond our borders.

Any church, synagogue, or major ministry can help you add someone's name to a prayer chain. Cancer survivors like me, who received daily prayers from countless unknown others, know the power of intercessory prayer. We

Time and again the Faith Principle plays a primary role in the healing of difficult or even so-called "impossible" cancer cases.

urge you to ask for that benefit which so many praying believers are ready and eager to provide.

I thank God for those who faithfully and consistently pray for the sick. Their prayers work. More often than we know, I believe they work miracles.

The Faith Principle

Time and again the Faith Principle plays a primary role in the healing of difficult or even so-called "impossible" cancer cases. Think of the Bible's rhetorical question: "Is anything too hard for God?"[2] We know there is nothing "too hard" for Him. Probably you know at least one "impossible cancer" that was healed. God never gives up on any of us. But do we give up on Him? And do we all too often give up far too soon?

When dealing with faith and healing, I believe there are some important caveats to consider:

1. Faith and medicine work hand in hand. *Never should one replace the other.* By faith, we seek guidance for our medical decisions. By faith, we enter into surgeries and other treatment with confidence. And by faith, we are guided to cooperate fully with the medical team working so hard to succeed on our behalf. Faith is *our* job; good medical practices, *the doctors'* jobs.

2. Faith is proactive. We *decide* to trust God with our health, our circumstances, our decisions, and our family. We *ask* Him to lead us through the cancer-treatment

process. We *choose* to trust God with the process and the outcome.

3. Faith in God, not faith in faith, becomes paramount. Mouthing words, ritual prayers, or mantras simply cannot substitute for honest conversation and intimate cooperation with the Lord God who created every cell in our bodies and each victory in our lives.

4. Faith causes us to respect the magnificent gifts of medical science. Knowing, as the Bible teaches, that "every good gift and every perfect gift comes from the Father above,"[3] we can accept even difficult medical procedures without anger, hopelessness, and rebellion, but with gratitude, confidence, and thanks.

5. It may be that we "walk through the valley of the shadow of death" during our cancer experience. But remember, we are just *walking through,* not *dwelling in,* and we need to "fear no evil." As the psalmist so beautifully proclaimed, "Thou art with me."[4]

6. But sometimes God says no to even the most fervent, faith-filled prayers. Though medicine does not always cure cancer, nevertheless, God always heals the believer—the total person—in so many ways. He also heals the hurting hearts of those who prayed so earnestly and faithfully for their loved one's survival.

When survival is not His answer, does that mean medicine has failed us? Did our faith prove fruitless? Was God indifferent to our pleas? Absolutely not! God holds in His

6

Those who place
their faith in
Him see many
marvelous
forms of
healing.

hands everything about our birth, our life, and our death. Those who place their faith in Him see many marvelous forms of healing: release from anger, unforgiveness or other sins, freedom from fear and pain, emotional healing, freedom within one's mind, healing of relationships, past mistakes, human regrets, and much, much more.

Nancy's Aunt Myra (names changed) wanted Nancy to visit her in the hospital and help address her Christmas cards. Aunt Myra, propped up on pillows, chatted as Nancy painted her aunt's fingernails and brushed her hair, being careful not to disturb the surgical collar around her fragile neck.

Though cancer had invaded Myra's brain, she spoke with energy and humor, directing Nancy to wrap and tag presents, which she had purchased well before the holiday season.

To the casual observer, this would have appeared to be an ordinary hospital visit. Myra's physicians and the hospital staff, however, found it amazing. With cancer throughout her body, including her neck and spine, how could she sit? How could she eat even soft foods when her throat should have felt sore from such intense radiation therapy? How could she be so alert and lucid?

There were no satisfactory medical explanations. The woman who giggled, chatted, issued instructions, ate, and enjoyed a manicure and a little family gossip had received no pain medications because she had no pain. Three days after that visit, her family Christmas preparations complete,

Nancy's Aunt Myra painlessly slipped away in her sleep, perfectly ready to celebrate an early Christmas with her Lord in heaven.

We all know that with cancer, medical cures do not always occur. Loss indeed can happen, and we may not understand why. But to "those who love the Lord and are called according to His purposes,"[5] healing, joy, and often an amazing enlargement of the spirit eventually come. We celebrate our beloved patient's life, understanding that God's plan for him or her is perfect. Nor is our precious friend ever lost, because we know exactly where he or she now enjoys perfect healing and perfect life.

As our human feelings of pain and loss subside, we can celebrate the one we continue to love, and celebrate even more the God who created and also loved that special person. I cannot imagine going through a cancer experience without the presence of God beside me. Fortunately, we need not try. He will walk with us every step of the way.

Spiritual Resources

I have talked with hundreds, probably thousands, of cancer patients during the past fifteen years. Some still feel shock from their cancer diagnosis. Others show fatigue from long months of treatments. Some are confident, others frightened. Whatever the physical or emotional state, however, I always ask whether they believe in God and believe He will help them.

HINT

I always ask whether they believe in God and believe He will help them.

Surprisingly, no one asked me that question when I was fighting cancer. Of course, Glenn and I attend church regularly. Both of us come from strong Christian families. My hospital room following my surgery was filled with friends who came to pray for me and for my recovery. Pastors visited, and noted evangelists telephoned to offer prayers and encouragement.

I relate all that to make a point: in the end, the only thing that really mattered was Dee Simmons' relationship with God. How much would I trust Him in that serious and frightening circumstance? Had I become indifferent to His presence in my life? Had I unwittingly moved away from Him because I was so busy? And was He still as real to me, as accessible and beloved, as my own husband?

I meet some people who have never considered God or made a place for Him in their life. Others intend to think about their spiritual life later, when they have more time. Still others feel their cancer is due to some divine judgment or punishment for earlier sins. And then there are those who, for some reason now feeling bitter and estranged, are no longer on speaking terms with Him.

The cancer appears. Life and death issues arise. *Is God the least bit interested in us when we have shown so little interest in Him?*

The Short Answer: YES!

Speak to God as simply and naturally as you would to anyone else. Tell Him how you feel. It's okay to complain.

Tell Him what you need. Confess your fears, anxieties, grief, or anger. We need not be the theological equivalent of a rocket scientist to get through to God. He knows us by name. Simply begin a conversation with Him and allow a divine friendship to develop between Father and child. This is a great gift, one many cancer survivors come to joyfully cherish.

The closeness that developed between me and God as I recovered from cancer surgery redefined my life and ultimately led me into meaningful new directions. Time and again I hear others say, as I do, "If it took cancer to make such wonderful changes in my life...." Yes, it was worth it!

So often cancer itself becomes the catalyst which propels us into an awesome appreciation of all we once took for granted. We see God's magnificent redemptive power in ourselves, our lives, and our family. Our only job is to allow Him into our life and present situation and trust Him with all we are and all we are facing. Say yes to God. Talk to Him about everything. If you keep those conversations private, that's fine. But if you share your interest in faith with your spouse, pastor, doctor, or friend, you'll receive some encouraging feedback.

Say yes to God. Talk to Him about everything.

Doctors are wonderful. I love my physicians and am grateful to them for all their knowledge, expertise, and care. They have blessed me for many years. But there is so much more for us to receive than even the finest physicians can give, and most doctors know that. "I can give you my best medical practice, but only God can heal," doctors say.

We all want the finest cancer treatments today's medicine can provide. But even more important are the seven thousand promises from God to us found in the Holy Bible. God's promises to mankind remain forever true.

The trust factor played an even more dramatic role in the lives of Harry and Cheryl Salem of Tulsa, Oklahoma, when an inoperable brain tumor attacked Gabrielle, the youngest of their three children and their only daughter.

Though the news hit the Salem family as hard as you'd expect, they did not cave in to fear. Harry and Cheryl Salem are known throughout the country for their Christian ministry. Earlier in her life, the then Cheryl Prewitt was crowned "Miss America" and had the privilege of telling audiences nationwide her own compelling story of the childhood automobile accident which left her leg badly broken and, once healed, considerably shortened.

The determined youngster began to pray that God would lengthen her leg, heal her limp, and allow her to become Miss America. The child's faith and dreams were rewarded, and Cheryl gave God all the glory. People across America found themselves profoundly touched by Cheryl's beauty and faith in God.

The faith only grew as she entered adulthood, ministry, and eventually into marriage with a man who shared her spiritual values and sense of mission. For the past twenty years, Harry and Cheryl, have ministered to thousands, particularly in the realm of healing. The couple understands much about the healing power of God and about our personal role in the process. If any two parents in the world could be said to have been especially prepared for Gabrielle's frightening diagnosis, they were the two.

"Doctors gave us two months and no hope," Cheryl told me. "But we had every hope, and we received eleven months."

Prayers for Gabrielle poured in from every part of the globe. Love reached out to her from every quarter. The faith-filled thoughts and efforts of countless thousands of believers surrounded the beautiful and much-loved child, yet the exhausted and heartbroken parents and her other siblings, Harry and Roman, at last had to relinquish her to their loving God.

Three months to the day after Gabrielle went home to heaven, Cheryl was diagnosed with colon cancer. She had experienced fierce bouts of nausea and profuse sweating for some time but would battle them off, attributing her symptoms to exhaustion following the family's eleven-month, non-stop battle in behalf of Gabrielle.

"I wanted to go home to heaven," Cheryl said. "I was used to fighting for myself; I've had painful fibromyalgia, horrible depressions, and chronic fatigue syndrome. But now I just wanted to go home. This seemed the perfect opportunity. I was so tired."

But she overlooked one important fact. "Our family was still in warfare mode," she said. Diagnosed on a Monday afternoon, Cheryl underwent surgery early the following Wednesday. Her desire "just to leave" meanwhile got pushed aside as she began considering her sons, their needs, and her desires for them.

About to be wheeled into surgery, under heavy medication, Cheryl opened one eye, looked up at Harry, and declared, "I'm not leaving you." As she explained, "I knew I was going to stay because I was going to be obedient to God. We had sons to raise."

"People so often don't realize they have a role to play in their healing," she continued. "Their attitudes, their hearts, their position in God.... Even really sick people can sustain hope and live for years past all expectations."

"But I didn't want to face what was coming with my cancer. I knew it would not be easy. I have no fear; I didn't like it, but I didn't fear it either."

After eight days in the intensive care unit, and time for recuperation, the exhausted wife and mother survived colon cancer. She underwent no adjunctive radiation or chemotherapy, embarking instead upon a regimen of vitamins, protein drinks, and other nutrients, with checkups every three months.

Today, Cheryl Salem says her immune system is strong. She has returned full strength to active ministry with its strenuous schedule of speaking, singing, and traveling. She knows she has much to share with others about God and His saving power to heal even the most sick and exhausted of His children.

I asked Cheryl how she would advise others to approach their cancer challenge. "Pray immediately," she advised.

6

"People so often don't realize they have a role to play in their healing."

"This will often offset any natural fears. Share everything with your spouse, every aspect of it. Harry did not leave my side for eight days and nights following my surgery."

"Speak out of your mouth whatever God has said to you. Read Matthew 18:18-19—and believe it. My whole life has focused on speaking God's words. I believe my battle was won because there was no fear. And God ordained for me to stay here a little while longer."

The little girl who suffered the terribly fractured leg and some one hundred and fifty stitches in her face became the teenager who prayed for her scars to vanish and her leg to become normal. Her Miss America crown serves as a glittering tribute to the God who does all things well.

Cheryl Salem today feels neither bitterness nor anguish about all that cancer has cost her family. There are no tormenting questions in her mind or in the mind of her husband. "Why?" we ask. "Why should heartbreak strike the lives of men and women who are so committed to God and live by faith in Him?"

Cheryl says she heard God's answer in her heart. "Because I can trust you. Because you can take it. Because you will teach others how to overcome." At age forty-three, Cheryl has faced many battles. With God, she and Harry have long ago learned to trust and not fear. "I look to the things that are eternal, rather than the circumstances of this moment."

Faith and Discipline

Faith like Cheryl's means that one has decided to be willing to follow directions and proactive godly self-discipline. It requires a day-to-day walk, ever alert to God's instructions.

Faith swings into action with regular prayer disciplines. "Not just daily prayer, but prayer as I go through each hour of the day," one man explained. "I talk to God about everything. Not formal, ritualistic prayers, but honest conversation with God should be the aim, and learning to listen for His answers to our questions and needs."

Faith swings into action with regular prayer disciplines.

How do we hear His answers? Those who pray soon learn that God may answer us via truths from His Holy Scripture, through circumstances, by words spoken by a godly friend, or by that silent but unmistakable voice which speaks to us in our heart. He always answers. Sometimes, however, we fail to listen.

A very intellectual and highly successful man I know once explained to me how he came to know and love the Holy Bible. Alone in a hospital room and facing cancer surgery within hours, the restless patient groped in a drawer of his bedside table and found a copy of the Holy Bible.

"I had never bothered to read it since childhood Sunday school days," he told me. "I had read many, many other books, but not this one." Now alone and feeling curiously depressed and empty, he picked up the somewhat battered volume and began reading passages at random.

"Why doesn't *everyone* read this book?" he now asked me in real amazement. "The power! The scope! I literally could not make myself put the book down."

His story is repeated again and again by millions of others who take up "The Book" and find it changes their lives forever. But many millions of others, equally needy, fail to explore its wonderful truths. They never realize that the Bible is God's love letter, signed in the divine blood of Jesus Christ, and written to each one of His hurting sons and daughters, including you and me.

The German theologian Dietrich Bonhoeffer, imprisoned and martyred for his faith by the Nazis during World War II, called the Book of Psalms the "prayer book of the Bible." I commend it, with all the other mighty books of the Holy Bible, to each of us during both times of distress and times of joy. Few physicians would fail to agree with my prescription!

Faith To Fight Cancer

Remember, the "measure of faith" was implanted in your being as you were created. You have faith already, and you can increase the faith you have. Remember:

- We serve a mighty God.

- He will never leave you or forsake you.

- He loves you with an everlasting love.

- He will guide you with His eye.

- He is able.[6]

REMEMBER

- We serve a mighty God.
- He will never leave you or forsake you.
- He loves you with an everlasting love.
- He will guide you with His eye.
- He is able.

Though this chapter on faith and healing has emphasized faith far more than medicine, survivors urge you to prayerfully and respectfully consider each. The gifts of today's modern cancer treatments are mighty. The gifts of faith within our individual lives are precious today, and they last through eternity.

The Faith Principle leads us to seek God with all our heart and wait expectantly for His healing of our bodies and our lives.

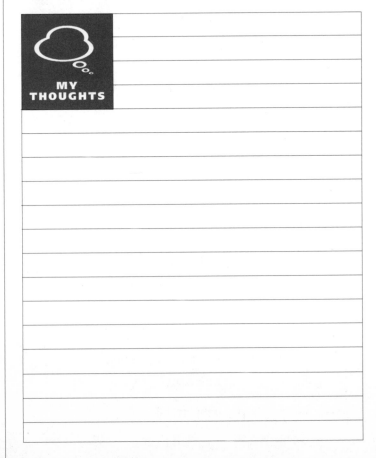

MY THOUGHTS

Principle 6
Adopt Faith, Hope, and Optimism

The decision to live life from a position of faith, positively affects healing and wellness, as many scientific studies show. Medical practitioners generally acknowledge the role of faith in healing. And clinical studies prove the remarkable results of prayer, hope, and an optimistic outlook.

Hope enables us to envision our healing. Optimism helps us expect and focus on success. Faith strengthens the inner person as we learn to trust God and expect Him to provide specific personal needs.

Result: The faith walk, which begins with a baby step, teaches us to live not as a victim, but as an overcomer. Faith promotes better recovery, reduced stress, lower blood pressure, good metal health, and even longer life.

MY THOUGHTS

MAXIMIZE LIFE

When cyclist Lance Armstrong's image appears on a television screen, you see a fit and smiling young father who obviously bursts with pride and delight as he looks at his adorable blonde son.

You would never guess that the superbly conditioned Armstrong, a three-time winner of the world-famous Tour de France bicycle race, only recently conquered cancer. Nor could you imagine that Destinae Rae, who recently sang to overflow crowds at the Olympic Games in Australia, is the same woman who fought through two bouts of breast cancer, treated not only with radiation and chemotherapy, but fourteen surgeries.

Walk down any busy American street or into any crowded office complex and you see others like Lance and Destinae: healthy and energetic, attractive, busy, and successful—and a cancer survivor. There are hundreds of thousands of us in America today, and the numbers steadily increase. According to the American Cancer Society, the rate of successful cancer cures continues to climb. One reason for that, in my opinion, is that cancers are openly talked about today, leading most of us to seek very aggressively the information, help, treatments, comfort, and solutions we need to fight the enemy intelligently.

Above all, we learn to maximize life. We give ourselves the best breaks possible during each day of our treatment process, and we continue that perspective in the months and years following our cure. In other words, cancer teaches us to respect ourselves deeply and to maximize our chances to live a wonderfully fulfilling life.

Parallel Universes

Cancer creates a temporary parallel universe for those who encounter it. There's the new Oncology Universe we enter, compared to the Old Familiar Universe we've occupied until cancer struck.

As we gather inner resources to fight cancer, we are also creating our personal blueprint for post-cancer success.

This provides a funny paradox: The seven principles which enable us to survive the Oncology Universe actually become the principles which lift us to additional success in our Old Familiar Universe. As we gather inner resources to fight cancer, we are also creating our personal blueprint for post-cancer success.

In other words, cancer itself can teach us some valuable ways to maximize life. This outlook can commence as we approach our cancer treatment journey and help propel us into new avenues of living that will enrich us forever.

Take a look at the seven principles that help us overcome cancer:

1. Take charge.

2. Get all the facts.

3. Strive for optimum health.

4. Boost your immune defenses.

5. Love more.

6. Adopt faith, love, and optimism.

7. Maximize life.

What Survivors Know

Survival secrets of those who surmount even intractable cancers or other vicious diseases seem to spring from an individual innate ability to maximize every life force he or she possesses.

As we wage all-out war on our particular cancer, not only do we practice some intense survival tactics, but at the same time we also adopt strategies for maximizing each day of our present and future life. Day by day, we learn how to make more moments become special. We learn the importance of *being* rather than *doing*. And many of us learn how to let go and allow ourselves to fall more deeply in love with others, and with our own unique life.

How, exactly, does one maximize life? It takes thought, decisions, and effort. Example: The simple decision to smile at each person who attends you produces fewer tensions, releases endorphins, and produces relaxation and feelings of well-being. As you know, that one small decision could effect positive changes in your happiness level and thus boost your immune system.

Such small but habitual life-affirming decisions put us in charge. You decide how you will control your cancer and your life. That one factor alone could make all the difference. Example: Following surgery, Emma asked her husband to bring her a rose, "a bud with tightly closed petals." The flower was sent up from the hospital's floral shop immediately, and during the next several days, Emma concentrated on its beauty and fragrance as she watched the blossom slowly unfurl.

The point is to choose where we will place our attention. As God tells us in the Old Testament, "I have set before you life and death. Now, therefore, choose life."[1] Today is a great day, despite even cancer, to decide to maximize everything about your life and all its potential.

I collect good ideas from experts on cancer survival, the survivors themselves. If you enjoy practical suggestions as much as I do, read this random list of good ideas from those who tried them and won. These potent quotes could produce

HINT

Moral: Instead of focusing on medications, wrinkled bedsheets, or other post-op discomforts, choose to occupy your mind with the wonder of something that gives you true pleasure; in Emma's case, one rosebud, but for you, perhaps a familiar book of poems, a light spritz of scent for your pillowcases, or a CD of happy show tunes.

some healthy new approaches to your present needs and lifestyle.

1. Put more happiness into your life. Do it now.

2. See your loved ones through new eyes. Appreciate them.

3. Laughter protects your sanity.

4. Find role models. It is easy to find others who have successfully coped.

5. Develop a sense of wonder.

6. Express your feelings. Say the words. Write the note.

7. Why should I have to be seriously ill before I can give myself permission to unwind?

8. Learn how to nurture and encourage others. Yes, even while you are the patient!

9. Resolve to possess a fully lived life.

10. Creative pursuits nurture the soul. Buy yourself a piano, an easel, or a new sewing machine.

11. Ask yourself daily: How can I take better care of myself? What health and lifestyle issues am I ignoring?

12. I choose to be happy.

13. God loves me exactly the way I am.[2]

14. I am not a victim.

15. I can create a happy new life.

16. I can confide in someone. He or she can confide in me.

17. Spouse: You are the person most important to his or her recovery. Do not neglect yourself.

18. I will give more of myself to others: time, advice, attention, affection, and encouragement.

19. Be honest about your needs. Be honest with yourself and others.

20. Negative self-talk is very damaging.

21. What, exactly, am I afraid of? Deal with it.

22. If God be for me, who can be against me?[3]

23. If you can't sleep, pray for others. Keep a list of names and needs. Check them off as prayers are answered.

24. Make specific plans for the future: start a business, paint the house, or throw a party. Set dates for each goal.

25. Write two or three thank-you notes each day. Keep plenty of writing supplies handy.

26. Surprise your nurse with a flower, a candy bar, or a sincere compliment. Nurses are overworked. Make their day!

27. Count your blessings daily—sometimes hourly.

28. Think of ways for your children to help you. Realize how much they desire to become part of your success.

29. My sense of humor always prevails.

I could go on. Actually, we could fill a book with similar cancer-inspired wisdom, and I'd like to urge you to do just that. Keep a small notebook handy and jot down the wise, sentimental, and humorous things people say about cancer, challenges, jokes, doctors, life in general, and you in particular. You'll enjoy reading those words some day. In fact, I'll go even further: a period of bed rest, recuperation, and going off line may inspire new avenues of creativity you never knew you had. One woman wrote deeply personal poems throughout the months of her breast cancer fight. She was amazed at the power of her writing. "I'd never written anything before except office reports," she said. Several years later, now fully recovered and fully occupied as a wife, soccer mom, and high-level corporate executive, she no longer has time to write for pleasure. Her newly discovered talent, however, is one she plans to pursue during a future season of her life.

Cancer experiences often reveal such personal clues, which can open life wider and add unexpected reward and adventure. Don't wait for some better time to begin trying new things, however. Do it now. Live your present life to the max.

I am struck with how often cancer survivors tell me about using the down time their illness provides. Instead of fuming about what they can't do, they make plans, explore ideas, or even begin new projects. These sorts of people do not allow cancer to take over their life but work around it. Serious illness, pain, or discomfort never completely derails them, because such people tend to consider their physical weakness merely temporary.

Destinae Rae was one who thought like that. As we mentioned earlier, she planned an extensive singing ministry,

TO-DO

Keep a small notebook handy and jot down the wise, sentimental, and humorous things people say about cancer, challenges, jokes, doctors, life in general, and you in particular. You'll enjoy reading those words some day.

CDs, a website, and other ideas and began to put her dreams into motion even before achieving a cancer cure.

Soon after learning of his well-advanced prostate cancer, Michael Milken established a foundation to foster medical research and public information about the cancer so common to the male population. Though his own prognosis appeared poor, Milken plunged ahead. Today the Foundation for the Cure of Cancer of the Prostate (CaP CURE), which Milken founded in 1993 and still chairs, is known worldwide for significant contributions to medical research and informing thousands of individual cancer patients and families about the disease.

In his website message about CaP CURE, Michael Milken explains, "We approach the problem of prostate cancer as we would a problem in business. Each year $100 billion is spent in the United States caring for people with cancer. Of this, only a small percentage is spent on finding a cure; the bulk is spent on cancer care. Is there an example anywhere in private industry of a company that would spend thirty times as much money to deal with a problem as it would to solve the problem? It just doesn't make sense."

Those are only two of the many cancer survivors I know about whose desire to serve others transcended even their own immediate personal health crisis. Dick Howe, after the then-new PSA test revealed his prostate cancer, immediately sent nearly two thousand letters to friends, relatives, and other executives, names retrieved from his business files. He informed them of his cancer diagnosis, told them about the simple test which had alerted him, and urged each male to seek a PSA test. Many who did discovered they had the disease.

Tom Redmond, another executive who appeared to be the picture of health and fitness when his cancer was recognized, also spreads the word about the importance of the PSA test. He has placed advertisements in national magazines urging others to seek regular PSA tests in order to catch the disease at its earliest stage, even before symptoms appear.

The creative individuals mentioned here allowed their personal cancer challenges to propel them into helping others—thousands, even millions, of others. These survivors not only involve themselves with other cancer patients, families, physicians, and medical research efforts, but the fascinating fact is that they all began their projects while battling their own cancer.

The thousands of men and women who have enlisted in clinical trials aimed at seeking better cancer treatments also are, in my opinion, the unsung heroes of the cancer war. Whether or not we should join such research projects remains a highly individual decision, one only the patient can make. These facts about clinical drug trials are basic to that decision.

A clinical trial is a research study to learn specific answers regarding new therapies, vaccines, or new ways of approaching known treatments. Carefully conducted trials determine the fastest and safest methodologies, and are both safe and effective. Only after laboratory and animal studies show promising results are clinical trials tested on people.

Ask your doctor if there is a trial he or she would suggest as appropriate to you and your disease. Ask how long the study will take, where it will be conducted, what possible side effects could ensue, and what possible benefits you might receive.

You'll also want to know who sponsors the study, what sorts of tests or procedures it might entail, and how it compares to other treatment options. Some clinical trials pay participants to join, while others do not. It is also important to note that participants can leave a trial whenever they wish.

Your physician will gladly provide candid opinions about the feasibility of entering a clinical trial in your particular case. If you prefer to stick to known treatments, that's perfectly understandable. But if you decide to join a clinical trial, you may receive new drugs and procedures that place you ahead of the current medical curve. The fact that you are helping advance medical knowledge can also provide intense personal satisfaction.

Trial participants are in no way "guinea pigs," but they are carefully monitored patients whose well-being and eventual success receive the utmost in care and management throughout the project and often well beyond. Medical science and the rest of us owe a huge debt of gratitude to the thousands of trial participants who have enabled the profession to advance to its present level, step by careful step.

REMEMBER

Your physician will gladly provide candid opinions about the feasibility of entering a clinical trial in your particular case.

Other Suggestions

A powerful weapon in our personal health arsenal is the information now so easily and quickly obtained. Major medical and research facilities spread the word about up-to-the-minute medical advances. Medical libraries, once largely off-limits to the public, now provide us with basic facts and the latest reports concerning health and disease.

Here's how to go about fact gathering:

- Learn the basics about your particular health or disease issue from a good medical dictionary or textbook at a library.

- Ask a medical librarian for help in locating medical journal articles and related information that you can print out.

- Computer users can get free access to medical journal references and abstracts from the National Library of Medicine databases through Pub Med at www.nchi.nlm.nih.gov.

- From your collected information, write questions to ask your doctor. Your own research might guide you to the best treatment options and facilities.

Remember that the internet and other research cannot replace your doctor. It is dangerous to self-diagnose and self-medicate. And while there's a wealth of solid medical and pharmaceutical information to be gleaned from the internet, at times the information proves contradictory or questionable. The Rand Group reports that nearly one hundred million Americans consulted internet sites for health-information last year.[4]

Carefully consider your sources. Be careful with the websites you visit and make sure you are comfortable with their privacy policies. Give personal information to sites you trust. Remember, too, that office internet searches could reveal personal information you'd rather not share with coworkers.

Virtually every cancer survivor I know comes to respect the life-and-death importance of boosting his or her immune system in every possible way. Afraid your cancer might recur? Instead of worrying, take steps to increase your body's built-in defenses. Of course we know our immune system needs all-out protection while we fight cancer, but any of us who experience this disease should make it a priority to become immune-system-aware for life.

One way is to isolate the elements in our life that we know in our heart of hearts to be detrimental to our health. Are you a night owl? A late-night TV junkie? Check out the role good sleep habits play in our immune system's operating capacity.

One of the most beneficial immune system boosters to adopt is that of getting eight hours of sleep each night. If you are wired for late hours, first read up on the importance of sleep. Then go shopping. Buy the new pillows, window shades, or whatever else you need to make your bedroom more sleep friendly. Make it a rule to reserve your boudoir for sleep and love-making only—no mystery thrillers, loud television, or work-related activities allowed.

Give yourself time to adapt to a longer sleep time, expanding it in thirty-minute doses and allowing your body's clock to adapt to the small changes. Find your natural sleep rhythm and begin to observe it. You might be surprised at how fast new floods of energy begin to pour in and how your face looks years younger. Note: More sleep = more energy = more effective and productive work. It does not hurt, either, that eight-hour sleep sessions often produce a sunnier disposition.

"Driven-ness" and exhaustion radically deplete the immune system. Adding more and better sleep to our life not only improves basic immune defenses, but puts more life into life, as well.

Far too many of us overlook the importance of good sleep habits for maintaining, a strong immune system, and here's another defense that's widely overlooked—emotional health.

Suppose American television and films were your main picture of our society. You'd probably conclude that we are a nation of rude, insulting, abrasive, violent savages. "Art" films often leave us feeling depressed. Too little of the material we watch lifts our mood or elevates our thinking, and too much of it leaves us feeling charged up, apathetic, or angry.

A new solution is to monitor our emotions and boost our health. We must watch all of our emotional input. There's no such thing as harmless or entertaining violence; ugly and

REMEMBER

One of the most beneficial immune system boosters to adopt is that of getting eight hours of sleep each night.

Note: More sleep = more energy = more effective and productive work.

inhuman images and horrifying sound effects assault our emotions and health.

But think about the last time you were isolated from news, radio, or television. Recall the serenity and simplicity of that time. Now imagine yourself free from all abusive emotional static. Imagine the healing balm pure silence provides. Imagine, too, the clear thinking and feelings of happiness you would enjoy. Perhaps these suggestions are mostly wishful thinking, but consider them as you seek ways to improve your immune system's functions.

Medical research has shown that adverse emotions lessen our immune system's ability to protect us. Noisy family arguments, feelings of resentment, and unforgiveness are destructive. We have the power to change negative feelings and adopt healthier attitudes.

Negative thinking such as pessimism and critical self-talk is toxic, many researchers contest. Poor habits of self-control and emotional "seizures" can literally make us sick.

Stay aware of the immune system's needs, including a calm, stable emotional climate in which to work at upbuilding, undergirding, and protecting our general health. The Bible offers a perfect prescription: "Whatsoever things are just, whatsoever things are pure, whatsoever things are lovely, whatsoever things are of good report, think on these things." [5]

Remember that right thinking and healthy emotions powerfully enhance our physical health.

We have the power to change negative feelings and adopt healthier attitudes.

The idea of eating nine fruits and vegetables per day, as *Prevention* magazine advocated as an anti-cancer measure, might seem impossible at first, but it's actually an easy immunity booster to acquire.[6] One serving could be a six-ounce glass of orange juice at breakfast; a medium-size fruit; a cup of raw veggies; or one-quarter cup of dried fruits.

You probably find yourself far closer to that goal than you realize. Other immune system boosters include the ollowing: whole grains, soy products, low-fat foods, organic foods, fresh fish, low-fat dairy products, nuts, and always, plenty of water. This heart-healthy, energy-boosting regimen takes little thought, effort, or money for the tremendous health benefits it provides.

Choose the freshest, most natural foods you can find and add a carefully chosen good nutritional program. The American Cancer Society reports that one-third of all cancers can be prevented by lifestyle changes, with nutrition a top participant in the Good Health Race.[7]

Even ten minutes of mild exercise can improve immune functions, scientists say. You don't need to enter marathons to create endorphins, which result in better feelings of well-being and alleviate stress. Mere ten-minute exercise sessions—a walk around the block, sweeping the sidewalk, chopping weeds—surprisingly add much to your total health.

What's more, it's never too late for even confirmed couch potatoes to begin moving their muscles and enjoying the benefits. When you feel draggy or blue, take a walk with

TO-DO

Choose the freshest, most natural foods you can find and add a carefully chosen good nutritional program.

HINT

Even ten
minutes of
mild exercise
can improve
immune
functions.

the dog or a grandchild, mop the kitchen, or turn on the radio and dance. Walk to the corner and mail a letter. Climb one or two flights of stairs. Whenever you make your heart pump and your blood run faster, you are doing good things for your muscles and your mood, your blood pressure and heart, and actually doing more good than most of us realize for the immune system.

Some ninety-year-old, wheelchair-bound nursing home residents have shown that lifting two-pound weights improves heart, lung, and muscle capacity. Few of us are too old or too weak to become at least a little more fit and toned!

Focusing on increasing our basic immune system by maximizing our general health obviously maximizes life itself. We become quite conscious of immune system defenses during our cancer battle, but most of us slide back into indifference and sloppy physical habits once we believe the war is won.

Whenever I speak to an audience, I make the same plea: *Improve your health.* As you can see, the project is simple. Good maintenance, such as most of us give our car, regular, reasonable habits, makes all the difference.

Once I heard a doctor advise his audience to take a personal health inventory once a year—not a doctor's exam, but a personal report card. Sleep? Nutrition? Exercise? Stress? Weight? Eye exam? Mammogram? And so on. Some items may be marked "NI"—needs improving. List the three that most need your attention and enter them in your databook. Immediately schedule an appointment for the dental exam, health club membership, or whatever your priority may be. By the time you complete item three, you are well on your way to significantly upgrading your health.

One important key to excellent health is consistent maintenance. We can find dozens of ways to improve immune functioning once we become aware, including such pleasurable pursuits as listening to music, climbing a mountain, or enjoying a massage. Be good to yourself all your life. Just do it!

A Life-Giving Spirit

The late Dr. Norman Vincent Peale, noted minister, author, and public speaker, often pointed out that the word *enthusiasm* comes from the Greek *en theos,* meaning "God within."[8]

No one can assess the power within any human spirit, but at those times when we see it shine from one of us like a bright flame, it awes and inspires the rest of us. When we add our small flame to the eternal glory of the Spirit of God, we begin to understand that such combined power actually at times produces miracles of healing. Many physicians have seen the enthusiasm, the "God within," that gives certain patients wonderful and inexplicable medical outcomes. Doctors may not be able to explain such things, but most acknowledge that they happen.

Increasing one's enthusiasm builds the human spirit and helps maximize life. Of course we can't promise that it will produce a medical miracle, but perhaps attaining a grateful

TO-DO

Sleep? Nutrition? Exercise? Stress? Weight? Eye exam? Mammogram? And so on. Some items may be marked "NI"—needs improving. List the three that most need your attention and enter them in your databook. Immediately schedule an appointment for the dental exam, health club membership, or whatever your priority may be.

REMEMBER

No one can assess the power within any human spirit, but at those times when we see it shine from one of us like a bright flame, it awes and inspires the rest of us.

heart and happy spirit is a miracle in itself. It is not easy to feel enthusiasm when plagued with chemo-induced nausea, fatigue, or mouth sores, but even despite all that, it can be done. How? By nourishing the spirit within us by all means possible. A cancer therapist says, "We feed our bodies, we educate our minds, but we neglect and starve our spirits. It's time clinicians begin to encourage patients to nourish their spiritual selves."

Whatever we focus upon will increase. At those times when we feel rotten, we might try to congratulate ourselves on another clinical session accomplished, another treatment milestone reached, or try to realize how fortunate we really are to be able to receive the excellent care available to us. By attempting to boost feelings of gratitude and accomplishment when the going gets rough, we mark another plus in our immune system column. We actively maximize life.

If nothing else, cancer teaches most of us the importance of beginning a discipline of tending our spiritual needs. Prayer and searching the Scriptures become vital elements in building up that part of us which will live on after this present life and survive gloriously throughout eternity.

Cancer teaches that even when humbled by present afflictions we can receive grace to learn more about such lifelong necessities as patience, love, tolerance, forgiveness, faith, acceptance, hope, and joy. Even on days when we cannot feel happy, we can feel joy.

If we allow it, cancer can also teach us how to cope with change. We begin to see that change is inevitable, for better

HINT

If nothing else, cancer teaches most of us the importance of beginning a discipline of tending our spiritual needs.

or for worse. To embrace change is to maximize life—physically, mentally, and spiritually.

True, such major changes as having cancer also mean major stresses: too many options, too many decisions, and too many challenges. The decision to find ways to strengthen ourselves spiritually at the times of overwhelming change can give us the faith, peace, and guidance we need to counteract stress overload and emerge stronger. The benefits and privileges of enjoying a disciplined and renewed spiritual life simply cannot be overstated.

Health may wane, fortunes may flounder, but our precious spiritual treasures need never dwindle or be lost. Our spirit is the one thing that can grow, increase, and prosper forever.

By faith we overcome not only cancer, but also any other evil that confronts us. By faith, we go from strength to strength. By faith, we build an ever stronger and more overcoming lifestyle.

Maximize life. Maximize your habits, health, wisdom, and wealth. Be filled with enthusiasm and the Spirit of God. These are the principles we cancer survivors have learned and for which we feel grateful.

May your own "walk through the fire," or that of your loved one, produce multiple healings and endless personal blessings as you learn how to minimize cancer's evils and maximize your greater life.

HINT

By faith we overcome not only cancer, but also any other evil that confronts us.

MY THOUGHTS

Principle 7
Maximize Life

Cancer, many survivors say, taught them to broaden, deepen, and continually celebrate life. They tell of mentally setting goals and making exciting plans for their lives, even as they were receiving chemotherapy.

Even at our lowest physical point, we can discover that it is possible to embrace life more fully than ever before. We can imagine ways to make ourselves and others happier; become more patient, tolerant, grateful, and kind; discover delight in slowing down and smelling the roses; express more love and affection; and help others in our home, our community, and our world.

Result: Serious illness and "down time" can lead us to larger, richer life experiences. Not only improved health, but more love, peace, gratitude, faith, joy, and service to others can arise from the ashes of the cancer challenge we face and overcome.

10 Ways To Put More Life Into Life

We survivors know how to celebrate. We enjoy life's tiniest nuances. Small events can become as important as great moments, and we allow ourselves adventures we might never have tried before facing cancer. Here are ten secrets most cancer survivors I know have learned about maximizing life.

1. Be honest. Face your circumstances, beliefs, and feelings squarely. Do not settle for less. Be transparent in your dealings with others.

2. Be grateful. You, more than most of the rest of the population, are keenly aware of the many blessings in your life. Speak your gratitude aloud and watch others catch your enthusiasm for life and living.

3. Be responsible. For yourself, your health, your lifestyle, your family, and your community interactions. Keep your promises. Stand tall.

4. Become health-minded. Balance your life. Respect the basic health and strength of your mind, body, and spirit. Take care of the health you possess, appreciate it and guard it throughout all the years of your life.

5. Keep finding new sources of joy. Music or mountain climbing, the wisdom of children, the pleasures of painting, writing, or woodworking. Take time to experience more personal creativity and inner growth.

6. Inspire yourself. Aim higher. Seek out experts who can teach you new subjects and skills. Every day, resolve to be enthusiastic about the activities you choose.

7. Enjoy new horizons. Read books you've always meant to read. Travel to Spain or Peru or Russia. Try scuba diving, astronomy, or hiking the Appalachian Trail. Explore places where, on a clear day, it seems as if you could see forever.

8. Expand your relationships. With the old and young, become interested, involved, and available. Good friendships and human interactions not only enrich life, but may actually lengthen it!

9. Nurture your spirit. Give yourself time, space, and quietude for personal thought, reflection, and prayer. Invite family members to follow your example of being as well as doing.

10. Become bolder. Empower yourself. Your beliefs matter, and so do your dreams. Listen to yourself, and act on the issues most important to your life.

In the great words of Moses in Deuteronomy 30:19, "I have set before you life and death, blessing and cursing; therefore choose life." Choose the great gift of more life, abundant life, and learn to increase it with every day you live.

Endnotes

Chapter 1

[1] American Cancer Society, *Cancer Facts & Figures 2000,* p. 1.

[2] American Cancer Society, *Cancer Facts & Figures 2000*

Chapter 2

[1] Martin E.P. Seligman, Ph.D., *Learned Optimism.* Alfred A. Knopf, New York, 1991.

[2] Larry Dossey, M.D. *Reinventing Medicine: Beyond Mind-Body to a New Era of Healing.* San Francisco: Harper, 1999.

Chapter 4

[1] Bottom Line Personal, Boardroom Inc., Greenwich, CN, Vol. 22, No. 4, p. 2.

Chapter 5

[1] Dr. Norman Vincent Peale. *The Positive Principle Today.* New York: Fawcett Crest Books, 1983.

[2] Peale.

Chapter 6

[1] *A Cancer Journal for Clinicians,* Nov./Dec. 1999, p. 347.

[2] *Prevention,* Aug. 2000, p. 122.

[3] American Cancer Society, *Cancer Facts & Figures 2000.*

[4] American Cancer Society, *Cancer Facts & Figures 2000.*

Chapter 7

[1] Psalm 139:14

[2] James Gordon, M.D., Georgetown Medical School. *Bottom Line Personal,* April 1, 1996.

[3] Beth Ginsberg and Michael Milken. *The Taste for Living.* New York: Time Life, 1998.

[4] Beth Ginsberg and Michael Milken. *The Taste for Living World Cookbook.* New York: Time Life, 2000.

[5] Dr. Richard Rivlin, Memorial Sloan Kettering hospital, in televised interview with Barbara Walters, Sept. 18, 2000.

[6] *Harvard Women's Health Watch,* Vol. 3, No. 6, Feb. 1996.

Chapter 8

[1] We Survive Together, *Parade,* Oct. 8, 2000, p. 31.

[2] Freud and Diane Guernsey, edited by Janet Carlson, Dealing With Depression, *Town & Country*, p. 186.

[3] Freud and Diane Guernsey, edited by Janet Carlson, Dealing With Depression, *Town & Country*.

[4] *Women's Day*, March 12, 2001.

[5] Mark 16:18

Chapter 9

[1] Leviticus 19:18

[2] Matthew 22:39; Mark 12:31; Luke 10:27

Chapter 10

[1] 1 Corinthians 13:8

Chapter 11

[1] Ephesians 6:13-18

[2] Genesis 18:14

[3] James 1:17

[4] Psalm 23

[5] Romans 8:28

[6] Job 36:5; Hebrews 13:5; Jeremiah 31:3; Psalm 32:8; Daniel 3:17

Chapter 12

[1] Deuteronomy 30:19

[2] John 3:16; Romans 5:8

[3] Romans 8:31

[4] RAND, www.rand.org, Press Release: "Click With Care: New Study Spotlights Problems and Potholes in Health Information on the Internet," May 23, 2001.

[5] Philippians 4:8

[6] *Prevention,* March 2001.

[7] *CA A Cancer Journal for Clinicians,* A Journal of the American Cancer Society, Volume 49, No 6, Nov./Dec. 1999, p. 329, Lippincott, Williams and Wilkins, New York.

[8] Webster's New World College Dictionary, 1999, Fourth Ed., Macmillian USA.

About the Author

In 1987 Dee Simmons was diagnosed with breast cancer, an experience that changed her life's direction. Following the diagnosis and an eight-hour operation for a modified radical mastectomy, Dee became determined to take charge of her health and her life. Five years later her beloved mother was diagnosed with cancer and lived only four weeks. Dee's life became a mission of healing and a passion for counseling and educating others about cancer and their need for optimum nutrition.

Today, Dee Simmons serves as chairperson & CEO of Ultimate Living International, Inc., with representatives nationwide. She founded the fast-growing company to meet specific nutritional needs of the one in three Americans who must wage battle against cancer, as well as those persons interested in prevention. Join Ultimate Living International, Inc., at www.ultimateliving.com.

Dee hosts a nationwide daily nutritional program called *Health Views,* sponsored by the Cancer Treatment Centers of America in Tulsa. Dee has also hosted numerous nutrition-oriented television programs throughout the country, along with appearances on *Make Your Day Count, Something Good Tonight, Celebration, In His Presence, Among Friends, Hope Today, COPE, The 700 Club,* and the *Armstrong Williams Show.*

Dee Simmons serves on the board of Disciples of Trinity, a Dallas-based charity assisting terminal cancer patients, and the board of Regents of Oral Roberts University. Dee was also named National Spokesperson for Making Memories Breast Cancer Foundation in 1999. She was ordained as a minister in July 2000.

Dee Simmons is a resident of Dallas, Texas, who at the age of sixty is enjoying great health. She successfully manages her own company, and actively participates in the lives of her family, husband Glenn (corporate excecutive and community leader) and daughter D'Andra.

To contact Dee Simmons

write:

Dee Simmons

c/o Ultimate Living International, Inc.

P.O. Box 191326

Dallas, TX 75219

For more information on Ultimate Living's

nutritional supplements and skin care products,

contact us at:

(214) 220-1240

or

www.ultimateliving.com

**Additional copies of this book
are available from your local bookstore.**

HARRISON HOUSE
Tulsa, Oklahoma 74153

Additional Health and Healing Books Published by Harrison House

Be Healed in Jesus' Name
by Joyce Meyer

Divine Healing
by Norvel Hayes

Getting a Grip on the Basics of Health and Healing
by Beth Jones

God's Benefit: Healing
by Marilyn Hickey

God's Creative Power for Healing
by Charles Capps

God's Word for Your Healing
by Harrison House

Healing the Sick
by T.L. Osborn

How To Live and Not Die
by Norvel Hayes

One Hundred Divine Healing Facts
by T.L. Osborn

One Word From God Can Change Your Health
by Kenneth & Gloria Copeland

Prescription for a Miracle—Healing Devotional
by Mark Brazee

Spirit-Filled Pocket Bible on Healing
by Harrison House

The Battle of Life
by Jesse Duplantis

Walking Through a Miracle
by Mary Frances Varallo

When Healing Doesn't Come Easily
by Lynne Hammond

Dee Simmons is National Spokesperson

for

Making Memories Breast Cancer Foundation

Making Memories turns dreams into realities to create special and lasting moments for patients diagnosed with metastatic breast cancer and their families.

Whether sending a family to Disneyworld or planning a family reunion, Making Memories Breast Cancer Foundation is dedicated to fulfilling the wishes and dreams of breast cancer patients.

If you want to help make a lasting difference in someone's life, please join Making Memories in creating something that will live forever...a beautiful memory. Contact:

Making Memories Breast Cancer Foundation, Inc.

P.O. Box 92042

Portland, OR 97292-2042

(503)252-3955

or visit the website

www.makingmemories.org

The Harrison House Vision

Proclaiming the truth and the power

Of the Gospel of Jesus Christ

With excellence;

Challenging Christians to

Live victoriously,

Grow spiritually,

Know God intimately.